INTO THE DARKNESS

A Journey into Schizophrenia

DARREN SMITH

Copyright © 2021
DARREN SMITH
INTO THE DARKNESS
A Journey into Schizophrenia
All rights reserved.

No part of this publication may be reproduced, distributed, or transmitted in any form or by any means, including photocopying, recording, or other electronic or mechanical methods, without the prior written permission of the publisher, except in the case of brief quotations embodied in critical reviews and certain other non-commercial uses permitted by copyright law.

DARREN SMITH

Printed Worldwide
First Printing 2021
First Edition 2021
Second Printing 2023
Second Edition 2023

11 10 9 8 7 6 5 4 3 2

Cover designed by MiblArt.

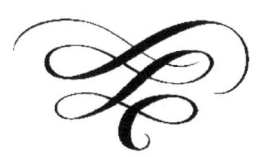

INTO THE DARKNESS

Dedication.

A big thank you to everyone throughout my life that went against the tide and stood by me, you know who you are. The ones brave enough to stand up and be counted. I could not have written this book without the loving support from my Wife Sam, who has put up with so much throughout the years and showing me that life has meaning.

I would like to dedicate this book to my late grandmother Rene Trendle and my very loving late mother Angela Allanson for never giving up on me. During those very dark moments that were life and death to me. No matter how torturous the journey was they never gave up. When nobody picked up the phone, my mum always did and I miss her dearly. I would like to thank my sister Jennine who helped me finance this project, without her I could never have afforded to self-publish.

To both my children Daniel and Joshua, thank you for your undying loyalty and love from you both. I am so proud of both of you, please do not follow my path.'

Prologue

As I looked at my compromised mobile phone, I knew I was under surveillance. The question was, did they want me to know, or had I found it by accident? Were they trying to make me go crazy again on purpose? Were they following my every move, filming and analysing me? As I drove up to the co-op, I looked in my rear-view mirror to see what cars were behind me. Was I being followed, or would they be waiting for me? I got out of the car and the voices hissed in my mind, 'They are always with him.' I decided that I would not hide but hold my head high, and if anyone were watching me, I would look at them.

Petrified, I walked in through the double sliding doors and looked around. Customers were milling around, but due to the pandemic, it was quiet. As I walked past the tills, a large middle-aged man glared at me. He knows, I thought, he is one of them watching me. The voices screamed in glee, 'He's seen one!' I gritted my teeth and forced a smile at him. He looked away in disgust.

My mind raced . . . how many of them would there be in the shop with me – five or six maybe? They would have a command centre close by monitoring my moves. I looked around at the customers' ears to see if I could see earpieces used in covert operations. The voices yelled obscenities at me as I walked around picking up my shopping, making snarky comments at me. People knew I was psychotic. They were talking about it amongst themselves. A young attractive blonde-haired woman looked at me as I walked up to the checkout. Was she one of them? I decided to smile at her to break the spell. She smiled back and my heart slowly stopped racing. As I paid the cashier, I was sweating and shaking, desperate to get back home.

After living with schizophrenia for the last thirty years, I have lived these moments hundreds of times over, and they never get any easier. I have gone into the darkness more times than I care to remember, but I always find my way back out. They say you cannot reach heaven unless you have visited hell first.

For all of you voice-hearers out there, do not hide in shame. Be proud of how strong and unique you are, and let's be more honest and open to stop the stigma.

If you or anyone close to you is suffering from related topics covered in this book, I would highly suggest you seek medical attention and be honest. Professionals cannot help you unless they know what is happening. There are so many support groups online now that you really are not alone anymore like I was.

Chapter One
My Childhood

I grew up in a small village in Buckinghamshire with two lovely younger sisters, Jennine and Melanie, and our mum and dad. We were not poor compared to some families, but we did not have everyday luxuries like biscuits, sweets, or crisps. Times were hard, so my dad worked three jobs to put food on the table, but at that age, you don't see these things. We were, however, lucky to have wealthy grandparents who had helped my parents out when buying our home. From what I understand, they gave my parents a sizable chunk for a deposit, and it meant they could buy their first house.

I have some memories of my first home in Buckinghamshire. It was a small terrace bungalow in a quiet cul-de-sac in a small town outside of High Wycombe. The children in the close were all friendly, and we would all race around the block on our bicycles.

After my youngest sister, Melanie, was born, we moved to Studley Green and lived in a three-bedroom bungalow with a lot of land. Studley Green was a small village on the A40 main road in Buckinghamshire. There was a school, a pub, and two little corner shops. Acres of fields and woods surrounded the area. My parents saved hard, and they renovated our home, building a lovely extension. During the renovation, my dad hired an expensive bricklayer to build a large ornate fireplace that spanned the width of our lounge. According to my dad, when it was complete, they stood back to admire the beautiful brickwork, crafted by a master tradesperson, and I turned to him and asked, 'Are you going to plaster it?' I was eight at the time.

The bricklayer stood aghast and fuming and said to my dad, 'Is he taking the fucking piss?'

My dad always laughs when he tells this story to me.

My sisters and I made our own entertainment. Jennine was only three years younger, and we would climb up our swings and slide, playing Batman and Robin. Wearing black Wellington boots was all I needed for my costume as I saved Robin, whom I made dangle off the ledge of the slide. Melanie was just a little too young to play with, but that did not stop her from trying to join in. We spent most of our time riding our bikes around the close and playing in the extensive garden. We had a few fruit trees, and I loved climbing them and gorging myself on the ripe plums. My best mate was a year younger than me and we did everything together. We used our imagination, like the time we found a toy ring and pretended we were hobbits. We took it in turns to hold the 'one' ring and would pretend to go invisible. The Night Riders hunted us on our way to Mordor, just like the hobbits. There were a lot of woods in Studley Green, and we knew them like the back of our hands. We hollered as we rode our bikes through them and built camps.

I remember my childhood Christmases like they were yesterday. My entire family met at my grandparents' house in Surrey. The house had three large double bedrooms: one was our grandparents' room, the second was the orange bedroom, and the third was the green room. The green room was the children's favourite room to sleep in – it really was the coolest. The garden was extensive, and my grandparents were fortunate to have an outside pool which we all enjoyed playing in during the nice weather.

It was a tradition every year: My whole family got together – my nan, grandad, great-grandmother (affectionately known as Big Fat Grandma), great uncles and aunts, uncles, aunts, and cousins. The day started with us opening presents and all the women fussing in the kitchen, preparing lunch. The men sat around chatting and the kids chased one another around, gobbling the Quality Street and Roses chocolates. As lunch got close, my grandad was called into the large kitchen and he sharpened his carving knife. He sliced the succulent large turkey and tender joint of beef, and the food was all laid out on the huge dining table, where we sat down to eat. All the adults sat at the large table and they put us kids wherever there was space. We pulled our crackers, donned our paper hats, and compared and traded the gifts, taking turns to tell our jokes. Then, in the afternoon, we played with our toys we got for Christmas.

We received our first home computer one Christmas in 1981, a Dragon 32. I plugged it into a spare TV in my grandparents' bedroom and played the one game it came with – *Berserkers*. We all knew some simple basic code from computer shops like Dixons Electricals, and we would make the screens blink 'Darren was here'. That evening, just like every other Christmas evening, my mum and uncles and aunts settled down with my grandad to play cards. Bets were small to begin with, but the cash soon piled up. The night went on as one by one, my uncles were gradually knocked out of the game, just leaving my grandad and mum. The atmosphere was electrifying and raucous as the drinks flowed. Long after we went to bed, my grandad was always beaten by my mum, and she would go home with a large amount of cash. It is only now, looking back, that I realise my mum was his favourite and he let her win.

My little school wasn't far from our home. It was incredibly quaint, with sixty children. I was more than happy walking there and back alone.

My class had such lovely children in it, and I remember one young girl asking me how old I was. I told her I was five, and she told me she was six and that that meant she was in charge. My time at little school was a happy one: they held regular events like school fairs and bonfire nights, all put on with the help of parents.

At nine, I left Mary Towerton School and started at Stokenchurch Primary School. I made friends very easily and have many fond memories of playing all the old-fashioned games like British bulldog, hopscotch, and kiss chase on the grass. One hot summer's day, while looking out of the window daydreaming, I saw the grass was being cut, and the smell was amazing; the sun shone into the classroom and I felt a gentle breeze on my face. It is just one of those fond memories that sticks in your mind and even now, every time I smell grass being cut, I am transported back to being nine years old again.

My favourite teacher was the deputy head, who was dreaded by everyone for his strict discipline. If you were naughty, he would give you two days to learn a long poem and make you recite it in class. I never met a kinder in all my life than Mr. Tidyman. During a parents' evening with him, he told my mum and dad that on many a dull day, I had brightened him up. He also told them he believed I would either end up as a future prime minister or a homeless tramp. When I was told this years later, it made me laugh and I smiled inside. In my last year of middle school, I sat my eleven plus. The 11+ was an exam to find out whether we were bright enough to go to an elite grammar school. Soon after, they gave us our results in envelopes and I sauntered home, opening my envelope on the way, only to read that I had failed. I had to walk home with sorrow in my heart about what my mum would say when I told her. I don't recall her reaction, so it could not have been awful.

I started at my local comprehensive school, Bartholomew Tippins in Stokenchurch, next to my middle school. The comprehensive school was equipped with a woodworking room, a large canteen, bustling classrooms, and a huge sports field. I cycled to school and back in all conditions. The road to school was a major A road with a national speed limit of sixty miles per hour. I would be shocked if parents today would allow this. But I never complained; I just got on with it. As I got older, I began cycling up to the library in Stokenchurch every Saturday afternoon. I spent many hours sitting in the small library, choosing books to read for the week. I loved sitting on my own, slowly reading the backs of all the old books, looking for stories that would interest me.

I was at my comprehensive for less than a year. I had a lot of friends there and no terrible memories of school. I was not academic, as my head was always in the clouds. After I'd been at the school for a couple of months, a fifth-year student, about the age of fifteen years old, approached me. His name was the same as mine, Darren Smith. He pulled me to one side one day and told me that people were out to 'get' anyone with our name and we had to watch each other's backs. I can't remember what I thought about him telling me this, apart from being confused, but looking back now, it was strange.

A few months later, my parents told me that my grandparents wanted me to go to a boys' private school and that they would pay. I did not question it and did as they asked me to do. It horrified me at how expensive it was, but I thought it was generous of my grandparents.

Chapter Two
Becketts School

My time at Becketts Private School was miserable from start to finish. There was nothing enjoyable at my new school. The lessons were strict, academic, and dull. I had one pleasant teacher, a young art teacher who was at least cheerful, but the other teachers were ridiculously strict, almost Victorian. My headmaster wore a long black gown and was feared by everyone. The school itself was an old large manor house set in extensive country grounds in Great Missenden in the Buckinghamshire countryside. The portraits of historical figures lining the halls and the large sweeping staircase to the first floor felt intimidating. Just being in the building seemed to suck the joy out of my soul. My classmates all came from wealthy families, so I stood out like a sore thumb. I remember in PE lessons, all my classmates had the latest sports bags, such as Puma and Adidas. My mum had made me a sack out of lilac fabric tied together at the top with a thick string. I felt embarrassed holding my kit bag and hoped nobody would comment on how poor I looked. I did not want to ask my parents for a new £30 sports bag, as I did not want them to struggle on my account. Some kids would boast about their families owning yachts or large companies, and some kids had motocross bikes, which they all took for granted. I dreamt of being able to ride a motocross bike over fields at the weekend. During political debate lessons, the entire class would all support right-wing parties, so just to piss them off, I would argue the merits of left-wing politics. In all honesty, I couldn't care less. I hated the fact they were all so entitled and seemed brainwashed by their parents. I would argue black was blue just to enjoy the pleasure of annoying them.

In my second year at Becketts School, things would take a terrible swing and my life would change forever. I was thirteen in 1982 and had just finished a piano lesson one afternoon when my mum collected me. It was a lovely warm day, with a slight breeze that felt pleasant as I walked to the car. We had an old bright-yellow Ford Escort Estate that we named Buttercup, and somehow, she just kept going. As I sat in the back seat, my mum told me she had to talk to me. I knew it was serious but was still not prepared when she told me that she and my dad were getting a divorce. I sat there stunned, like someone had slapped me across the face, not knowing what to say. She told me that there would be a family meeting on Thursday evening to discuss things. She said that she would like me to live with her when they separated. I had no favourite parent as a child; I loved them both but understood it was common for kids to live with their mothers after a divorce, so I agreed.

Thursday evening came around and my dad picked me up from my school coach on the back of his motorbike. As we pulled into our cul-de-sac, he told me we were about to talk about a divorce and that he wanted me to choose to stay with him. He said that my mum would change her mind about the divorce if I went to live with him. I was just thirteen years old, and they were putting me in the middle. I felt torn. I had no idea what to do but agreed with my dad in the hope they would reconcile.

The meeting was heart breaking for me, and at the meeting, they asked me who I would like to live with. It was an impossible decision but I believed that if I chose my dad, they would not split. My mother felt I had betrayed her; she didn't even realise why I had chosen my dad. I understand both sides of the story. I blame neither of my parents for anything that happened during this time. Both of my parents are good, loving, decent people; I love them dearly and I have no wish to hurt them.

I remember being on the school coach one morning; I was fourteen, and my heart broke in two. I can recall the anguish that I felt in my chest. The despair pulled at me, dragging me into depression, the loneliness and pain cutting into me. I didn't have many friends at school and certainly no close friends I could talk to. I was alone and in a desolate place. The school had been informed of the situation by my parents, and yet not one teacher came to me and asked if I was okay or if I would like to talk. At the time, I just wanted a hug from someone and to be told I would be okay, but it never came.

As time passed, I grew angry and did what any kid in my situation would do: I rebelled. I hung around with about six or seven classmates and we would walk down to the woods at the back of the school for a sneaky fag. On a couple of occasions, a horrible kid called TJ brought in some cannabis resin and we all tried it. I felt such guilt at trying drugs, but I don't remember feeling stoned. TJ came from a poor migrant family as a baby, and they had been lucky and won the football pools, investing their winnings into a chain of fast-food restaurants. His parents gave him bundles of cash whenever he asked. And he carried a rolled-up wad of £200 notes on him at all times. He was a spoiled kid, and large for his age. He would bring in wholesale boxes of chocolate bars, handing them out here and there. Over time, I realised he was a spoiled bully who had no friends, so he bought them. He would treat everyone to chocolate except me, and because he knew he could not buy me, he hated me.

Throughout my time in school, TJ bullied me, and all the groups we hung out with chose him over me. I was a bit too frightened to fight back, as we often fear bullies. One time, I threw him over my shoulder using judo, which I had done for quite a few years. But instead of piling into him whilst he was on the floor, fear pulled me back. One day during lunch break, TJ beat the crap out of me and the gang who had once been my friends taunted me whilst it happened. After the beating, we all headed to our classes and I sobbed and sobbed during the lesson. The classrooms were tiny, and our teacher never said a word to me. I always considered him to be a nice, respectable man and he was liked by all pupils. But it was impossible to miss me sobbing hard in a small room of eighteen pupils, and he ignored me and just continued teaching the class as if I were not there. I cannot understand why I was not taken out of the class, sat down, and asked what on earth was going on. It was cold, heartless, and unforgivable. I felt hollow inside, like I was no one, and I despised everyone in my life. I realised that life was cruel, and I began to think that compassion did not exist in any form.

My time at Becketts School became even more miserable, and there was bullying everywhere I looked. Another classmate, Dan, was verbally bullied, often being called 'gay'. I felt very sorry for him, and after a while we became friends. Dan's parents spoke to the school, but nothing was done, and he left to go elsewhere. He was a kind, caring, and good-looking boy. We shared the same taste in music and began hanging out in our local town, High Wycombe. There were the punks, skinheads, hip-hoppers, rockers, mods, and our choice: new romantics. We dressed like our pop idols, Duran Duran and Japan, with big hair and large shoulder pads. We lived our choice of fashion and music and would spend hours in the Our Price record store looking through the vinyl records. We made a lot of friends in High Wycombe. We would chat with anyone our age if they were friendly. Wycombe was a large market town with a big bustling shopping centre. During the weekends, the town was full of shoppers and teenagers dossing around. We would wander around the streets which would be heaving with people visiting their favourite shops. Our favourite hangout was the top-floor balcony of the shopping centre The Octagon. We felt that we belonged there. Every Saturday, we caught the bus for the forty-minute trip to Wycombe. I feel sorry for teenagers today; they never got to experience the joy of choosing a 'fashion.' It was fun and gave us a sense of belonging.

But my times in High Wycombe weren't always pleasant. One Saturday, a small group of us 'new romantics' were walking around when a group of skinheads decided to attack us. They were twelve people of mixed ages, some even adults, and we were outnumbered. Things turned very nasty and a big fight broke out. I have a brief memory of the incident, but a police sergeant came to help us and an older skinhead strangled him. I have no recollection of it all, which I now find odd because I remember an awful lot from my past, but it's blocked. I was asked to go to court as a witness and I would have declined, but the police sergeant had put his life in danger to protect me. I gave my name and address as I stood in court, frightened that the skinheads would now know my address and hunt me down. They were sentenced and some went to prison.

One evening, Dan, his pretty older sister, and I (being only fifteen at the time) pooled all of our money, getting together about £6.50 in silvers and coppers. We walked to his local off-licence and, being the ballsy one, I went in and walked up to the counter. I told the owner I wanted to buy my mum a bottle of whisky for her birthday and showed him my money. To my disbelief, I walked out with a bottle of Bells Whisky. We sat in the nearby park, and each of us took a good swig. I was able to drink it neat without a problem and I drank two-thirds of the bottle. That night, I remember being woken by a doctor in Dan's bedroom. Buckets of sick surrounded me, and the doctor asked me if I had been sick that night. I told him no as I vomited. I was so ill that Dan's parents had to call the doctor as an emergency, and they never ever told my parents. I also found out I kissed Dan's sister and it gave me a warm feeling inside, as I fancied her.

Chapter Three
Yvonne

When I was fifteen years old, during the summer holidays of 1984, I stayed at my other grandparents' house in Weston-Super-Mare in Somerset. The bustling town's beachfront was full of attractions. I walked down to the sea, and the sun shone all week, and I felt happy and carefree. It was at least an hour's walk from my grandparents,' but the scenery walking through the woods was lovely, so I enjoyed it. I was happy just to walk around the town and take in the sites and atmosphere. The beach was full of families enjoying themselves. The pier was full of attractions and rides, the latest pop music was playing through the Tannoy system, and it seemed magical.

One day, I was propped up against a wall on the promenade, taking the world in, when two girls the same age as me came up to me and we started chatting. It turned out that they lived close to me in Beaconsfield, and they, too, were staying at their nan's house. We hit it off, and within days, one of the girls, Yvonne, and I were a couple. Yvonne was medium height with shoulder-length brown hair. She wasn't particularly pretty but had a lively personality. Living close to Yvonne made seeing each other frequently quite easy. We spent most weekends together at either her mum's flat with her step dad or at mine. For the first time in years, I felt loved by somebody, and I cannot thank her enough for that, as I craved love and affection. Our relationship blossomed, and within a couple of weeks, we found ourselves in an empty field next to my local park. The inevitable happened, and we lost our virginities to each other.

We had no idea what sex was supposed to feel like, and I don't think I realised that sex with a virgin was nothing like normal sex. We met a week later at her father's house. He was out, but Yvonne's older sister was in. Her sister was seventeen, in college, and stunning looking. Yvonne and I went to her bedroom and began fooling around. Before we knew it, I had my first taste of sex. It was not loving . . . it was pure lust, and the most intense physical pleasure I had ever known. I hadn't believed in my wildest dreams that sex could be anywhere near as amazing as this was.

Yvonne and I dated for six months, and whilst there were a lot of love and affection between us, it was a very intense sexual relationship driven by an insatiable lust. Yvonne often wrote me long letters about what she wanted to do to me. Her notes were shocking and would put Fifty Shades of Grey to shame. One evening at her home, we became playful, and she tied me to her mum and stepfather's bed. Yvonne used her stepfather's work ties and bound my wrists and ankles, which I found quite unnerving. She left me tied up, naked, and disappeared to her kitchen to fetch something. When she returned, she sat atop my legs and put ice cubes in her mouth, crushed them up, then gave me a blow job. I am still lost for words now when I think back to this. We were only fifteen years old, and in all reality, children. As a typical fifteen-year-old boy, I told friends about our experiences. Word got around and I got a name for myself.

Yvonne's mum was pleasant, but her father and stepfather hated me. They warned me to never lay a hand on her. One weekend, my mum had to go in for an operation on her womb and we decided we would tell Yvonne's parents she was staying at mine for the weekend. We then told my mum that I would stay at Yvonne's. With my home empty for the weekend and no parents to keep us apart, we slept in my mum's double bed. My dad had moved out at this point. It did not even occur to me how disrespectful it was to have sex in your parents' bed. Whilst my mum was in the hospital, there was a serious complication and she had to have invasive surgery. She called Yvonne's mum and thanked her for looking after me whilst she was in the hospital, asking if they wouldn't mind having me for longer. Yvonne's mum told my mum we had been staying at mine and she knew nothing about her being away. . . . We were in trouble. The proverbial shit hit the fan. My mum came home and realised we had slept in her bed. She was furious with me, as were Yvonne's parents. I don't think they even knew what to do with us.

We visited Yvonne's dad a couple of weeks later and had lunch with him and Yvonne's hot older sister. During the meal, her sister played footsie under the table . . . but not with my feet. I made my excuses to go to the toilet as her foot caressed my groin. I never told Yvonne, as I did not want to break the trust that sisters share. I cannot to this day figure out if Yvonne's dad set her up to do this, or whether her sister was just horny as hell. A week later, I was at Yvonne's flat and her stepfather asked if he could have a word with me. I followed him out to the stairwell, and he put me up against the wall and told me they had warned me to never touch her. He questioned me and threatened to throw me over the stair balcony, telling me my judo would be useless against him. A week later, we were banned from seeing each other. I felt my heart had been torn out and cried all week. We were each other's first love, after all. A week later, a friend and I went to the cinema to watch a film, and I bumped into Yvonne. She was with a new boyfriend and I was fuming; I felt betrayed. All it took was a week to get over me and I vowed revenge.

Chapter Four
Crime

Wanting to hurt Yvonne as much as possible, I asked out her friend Cath. It was casual and did not last long. She was an attractive girl who was a bit shy, and we never slept together. During this time, there was a party being held in a hall next to a primary school. I attended it with my classmates and Cath, and we all got drunk. A couple of us decided stupidly to break into the school and cause damage. We tipped over tables and smashed a window. It was so mindless – a stupid thing to do, and I have no idea why I did it. I caused damage for no reason other than that I could. The police investigated the incident, and I was called in for an interview before being read my rights. I admitted what I had done and eventually received a warning and a fine, which I think my mum paid. It terrified me to be in so much trouble with the police and I felt helpless and so guilty. This was not the only time I broke the law, and looking back now, I am ashamed of my behaviour. I cannot fathom why I did the shitty things I did in my teenage years. All I can do now is look back and feel a deep sense of remorse for my actions and ask for forgiveness.

My mum began seeing a young guy named Adam. He was about twenty-five years old, one of our judo instructors, and an idiot who lived at home with his parents. There was nothing likable about him, and he was terrible with kids. All he was interested in was my mum. During a science lesson at school, our teacher introduced us to the dangerous chemical sodium. If taken out of the protective solution they kept it in, it was flammable. We were told that, if mixed with water, it would explode. Say no more. We stole the lot, and on the coach home, I got some small pieces out and spat on them as the sodium fizzled and sparked. When I got home, I called Adam outside, grabbed a bucket of water, and threw the sodium in. Within five seconds, the bucket flew in the air fifteen feet and exploded. He did not seem to be impressed and went inside. I called my sister, Jennine, into the bathroom, then laid the sodium out on a piece of toilet tissue, and filled the basin with water. As Jennine came in, I told her I was going to show her something cool. She looked over the basin, and her arm caught the toilet paper, knocking the sodium into the sink. I panicked, knowing what was going to happen. I darted for a towel to throw over the basin. Jennine decided she wanted to see what was going on with all the sparks and looked into the basin when bang, it exploded right in her face. Time slowed down as the explosion happened. Adam was in the bedroom with my mum and came running into the bathroom, where Jennine was on the floor crying and holding her face. I ran out, crapping myself.

My mum and Adam took Jennine to the hospital, where she had her eyes examined and washed out. It blinded her for two days, but her sight eventually came back. I felt so awful that I ran away. I got to a pub on the way to Marlow, trying to get to my dad's new flat. I called my school friend Richard, who told my mum and Adam where I was, and they came and picked me up. I should imagine the shit hit the fan at school, as I had stolen explosive materials from the unattended open school lab stockroom. My sister has now forgiven me, but occasionally it is mentioned that I nearly blinded her.

In my last year of school in 1985, after selling our bungalow, my mum moved to Surrey to be closer to my grandparents. I had about seven months left at school, and my exams were looming. One of my friends' parents offered to let me stay with them when my mum and sisters moved so I could finish my studies. It was a very kind gesture, and they were very good to me. Out of school, Richard and I dossed about as kids do, going to local discos in pubs and occasional house parties.

I had two horrible incidents whilst at those parties. As most teenagers do, they buy cheap alcohol and enjoy getting drunk. The first incident happened when I was paralytically drunk and a girl nicknamed 'The Barrel', because she was unattractive and as wide as she was tall, led me outside the party and propped me up the garage wall. She pulled down my trousers and gave me oral sex against my will. I was too drunk to even care, but the next day, I felt angry that she had taken advantage of me, as I would not have touched her with a ten-foot barge pole. The second incident affected me even worse. I was at another house party having fun and had drunk an entire bottle of Cinzano. A local girl called Marion asked me to go upstairs with her. I told her no; I was not at all interested. She took hold of me, and in my inebriated state she guided me upstairs to a bedroom. She laid me on a double bed and undressed me. Even though I was paralytic, I knew what she was doing and told her I did not wish to and said no. She forced herself on me, putting a condom on me, and I lay their shit-faced whilst she had her way with my near-comatose body. Even though I did not want sex with her under any circumstances and said no, I ejaculated . . . and even to this day, I feel confused about that. She climbed off me and realised that the condom had split. What she said to me next frightened the hell out of me. She told me that if she got pregnant, I would stand by her or 'she would get her Black mates on me.' The whole incident was awful, and for weeks I was worried her friends would lynch me. I have always wondered where this stood in terms of rape from a moral and legal point of view.

I was never close to Richard; he was more just company, and he was not a good influence on me. He told me he used to break into a local factory and explore and get up to mischief. Being the rebellious idiot I was, I soon joined him. Something happened at one point and Richard's father found evidence of our wrongdoing and contacted the owner. The owner took no action, but it was obvious that they had found us out. In hindsight, I am shocked that the police were not involved. I feel very guilty about the damage we did, smashing industrial light bulbs and letting a powder fire extinguisher off on the common.

During my time at Richard's, I was never asked about my parents' divorce or how I felt, even though I was dying inside, and Richard's parents never realised how traumatic it was for me. Richard had an air rifle and seemed obsessed with shooting squirrels, which he considered vermin. Every time he killed one, he would cut off the tail and hang it on a hook in his bedroom window. One day, he told me to try it, so I shot a pigeon in his garden, but it didn't kill the poor bird and I had to put it out of its misery. I felt a tremendous sense of guilt that I had killed a bird and vowed I would never, ever take a life again, no matter how small, unless it was for humane purposes.

My crime spree didn't happen regularly, but I did some very shameful things. I cannot figure out my reasons for these actions and I took no pleasure in any of it. We threw stones at a car window once, and I am now extremely ashamed that, at that time, I had no conscience. As I have grown older, I often ponder what goes through the mind of criminals and I cannot fathom their mindset. I wonder if they feel any guilt or pleasure in causing suffering, and also if they sleep easily at night, knowing how much suffering they cause. I would hazard a guess that they, like me when I was younger, have no empathy for those affected.

In the future, I would change and try my damnedest to live a clean, honest life, not only because it was the right thing to do, but I wanted a clean conscience. Following my decision to turn over a new leaf, I tried to live by a moral code of which I would be proud.

My last six months at Becketts became very chaotic, and most of my classmates, including me, were out of control. There is no better way of describing us except as feral little bastards who were hell-bent on causing mayhem with no thought of others. We taunted our teachers to the point where our poor art teacher walked out in tears. A very strict teacher taught us our RE class, and we decided that in our last lesson with him, I would take in a cassette recorder and record the lesson. Our plan was to disrupt the class as much as possible and cause mischief during the class. We had an empty Coke can and began throwing it at one another every time his back was turned, hoping the person they threw it at would not catch it and get in trouble. This happened when I threw it at Richard, and our teacher let loose. As he turned on Richard, who dropped the can, we all laughed. The teacher yelled at us and everyone stopped laughing, except me. I was in hysterics and ignored his wrath. He called me up to the front of the class in an absolute rage and told me that in all his time as a teacher, he had never wanted to punch a boy in the face as much as he did right then to me. Our tape of the class did the rounds, and we found it hilarious.

I can't remember if it ever came to light at the school, but afterwards, I was suspended and banned from classes. I spent the rest of my time confined to the old head teacher's office to study for my exams. The room was bare, with an enormous desk and a row of filing cabinets. Being the little bastard I was, I began looking through them and discovered that they contained files on every pupil and teacher at the school. I read my file, and that of one of our kinder teachers whom I respected. His report showed he was under a lot of pressure to improve his targets or he would face disciplinary action. I felt terrible for going through the files after reading that and stopped looking.

My exams were looming within a few weeks and boredom soon set in. During breaks, I could mix with the other pupils. A large kid, Matt, beat the crap out of me in the toilets at every opportunity he got. I never knew why, but, as before, I never stood up for myself, as I believed I wasn't strong enough.

Chapter Five
Surrey

I took my exams at Becketts, failed, and moved to Banstead in Surrey with my mum and my two sisters. I moved everything to my new home in Surrey, where I soon felt at home. The house had three bedrooms with my two sisters sharing; I had the box room. It was small but comfortable. We had a small garden and a large double garage which would become my sanctuary in later times. The evening I moved in, I explored the town. It had a homely feel to it, with a small but busy high street and three pubs. That evening, I walked down to the high street and met a small group of mixed kids. They were friendly, and I felt welcomed. As time passed, I mixed with the local teenagers, who would sit around chatting and making their own fun. They were a friendly bunch, and I felt very at home.

There was a large comprehensive school which my sisters attended, and they soon made lots of friends. The next town over was a huge council estate with their own secondary school, and it became clear the two groups did not mix and there was some rivalry between them. Because I attended neither of these schools, I was not seen by either side as a threat and was welcomed by both. Over the years, I made some excellent friends.

Within a week of my moving to Surrey, my mum marched me down to the local college, NESCOT in Ewell, and with no idea I wanted to do, I signed up for a basic construction diploma which gave a very broad but basic general knowledge of the industry. I made a few good friends in class and we would often meet at my house and walk to college. It was a good six-mile round trip to the college and coming home was uphill all the way. It didn't bother me in the slightest, and I have fond memories of enjoying my walks, especially when my best mate, Joe, joined me. During my year at college, it became clear that I had no interest in the subjects being taught and I would bunk off with Joe. We would hire a video and chill out at mine. The hub of college was the refectory, where there was a canteen and bar for mature students. It was so alive and thrilling. One guy in my course, George, and I would chat at break and lunchtimes. He would always buy a hot panini. He was very kindhearted to me and knew I was hungry, as I had little money. Every day, he would share his lunch with me, and I have never forgotten his genuine kindness. George was a big lad and was fortunate to work Saturdays and Sundays for a builder as a labourer and hod carrier. He was on a massive wage of £50 a day, which in 1985 was a small fortune for a seventeen- year-old. George and I became good friends; he used his mum's top-of-the-range Golf GTi, and we went out a lot to pubs, clubs, and parties.

At sixteen, I soon found work with my local Woolworths as a Saturday boy. All the staff were girls my age, barring the general manager, who was a bit of a boy, but good to me. I worked hard at Woolworths and it was a fun place. There were a lot of funny stories from working at Woolworths, but one of the funniest ones was when I bought a dodgy porno VHS cassette. There was a girl from a very well-to-do family who worked with us. She was nice and nobody disliked her, but a couple of us decided to prank her during her lunch. In the breakroom, there was a TV and video player, and I set it up so that as soon as she flicked it on, the porno would start playing. We picked a shocking scene and waited. When she entered the room with her lunch, she sat down and popped the TV on. I was hovering in the small kitchen to catch her reaction. Sure enough, the video began playing, and I saw Nina's face display sheer horror at what she saw. She was so flustered, she did not know what to do. Being the mischief-maker I was, I found it hilarious and went and told the rest of the staff about her reaction. In the future, as we got older, the story stuck, but not maliciously – more out of fun. I was sweeping the floor once when two girls in their twenties came in. One of them walked up to me and grabbed me between my legs and said, 'Show me your bits.' Her friend apologised and told me she wasn't well, and they walked out. It was odd. I earned a meagre £30 a week but somehow got by, even as a smoker.

Walking to college every day was tiring, and it took me an hour each way. My mum had found work locally and decided I would benefit from a moped. Kindly, she bought me one, and when it arrived, I did not have a clue how to ride it. The first time I took it out, I wobbled down the road, not knowing how to change gears or even brake. I ended up riding down a steep hill close to home and wound up in a hedge at thirty miles per hour. I was not hurt, but I am pleased that these days before you can even get on a bike, you must take a basic course at a local riding school. Within a week of having my moped, it went wrong. As with old two-stroke mopeds, they are very temperamental, and they need some basic mechanical knowledge just to keep them running. I broke down a couple of roads away and a guy a few years older than me came to my aid. Steve was a biker who had passed his test, and there was not much he did not know about fixing them. I would later meet his younger brother, Donald, and we would become close mates because of our love of motorbikes. As time went on, I learned how to ride, eventually buying a bigger, faster, and more reliable bike. A small group of us with a love of riding would hang out. Back in the day, bikes were restricted, but there were plenty of tricks to get around these restrictions, and it almost became a competition as to whose was the quickest bike. A few miles away was a very popular beauty spot called Box Hill with an enormous car park and a small cafe. Every Sunday, hundreds of bikers from miles away would meet up, chat, and admire some of the works of art. Some of my happiest memories are spending Sunday mornings polishing my bike and meeting up with the gang and chilling out, whilst riders would race up and down the dual carriageway and pull wheelies next to the car park. It seemed like every Sunday spent down at Box Hill was hot and sunny. At seventeen, we all thought we were Barry Sheen and damn right dangerous. It became a bit of a prank to ride up next to a mate and pull his keys out of the ignition and throw them in the road. His bike would stop, and he would have to retrieve his keys and catch up to us. One sunny Sunday, when a mate had his keys taken out and thrown on the road, he was going around a tight bend and the automatic steering lock came on. He ended up on a full left-hand lock and mounted the pavement, crashing into a hedge. He was incredibly lucky to come out unharmed, but it could have been fatal. We found it hilarious, but we stopped pulling each other's keys out after that.

Chapter Six
Jennifer

It was not long before I met a lovely girl called Jennifer. She was the same age as me and doing an animal care course. It was Valentine's Day, and she sent her friend over to me in the refectory with a card. It read I want to kiss and cuddle you. I looked over, and she was smiling at me. Jennifer had mousey short blonde hair, lovely blue eyes, and a pretty smile. Jennifer and I dated for maybe six or seven months. I would ride to her house occasionally on my motorbike. She lived on the other side of Guildford, near Cranleigh, and the journey would take a good hour, riding through country lanes. Every lunchtime at college, we would walk over the car park to a disused field. There was a large mound of earth blocking the view to the field, and nobody could see us. We took advantage of this every single day in college for six months, and our libidos never seemed satisfied. I remember one lunchtime, we ended up next to the car park and by the motorbike shed, lying on the grass. It was a gorgeous sunny day, and I lay back soaking in the warmth while Jennifer was giving me oral sex when we heard screeching tires. I looked up to see a bunch of my classmates jumped out of Joe's car. They were yelling and laughing and cheering me on. My classmates at the time thought I was a bit of a legend because of this. I remember feeling quite popular in college and that was quite new for me.

During this time, I became best friends with a girl named Jan who lived just up the road from me. I would spend a lot of time lying on her bed, chatting and listening to music. She was very intelligent, pretty, and had lovely long dark-brown hair and deep brown eyes. We shared the same stupid wacky humour. Nothing ever happened with Jan because I was with Jennifer, but I loved her as a friend. One evening while we were chilling at mine, my mum invited Jan over for Sunday dinner, which was about ten days away. I forgot about our Sunday roast plans, though, and on the Saturday before, I invited Jennifer over to mine on Sunday, arranging that her mum would drop her off at 3:00 p.m. The night before, my mum reminded me that Jan would be over for lunch and the penny dropped . . . Shit! Jan was due over, and in my mind, I figured I could get her gone in time for Jennifer at 3:00 p.m. I was a nervous man on Sunday morning but figured I could pull it off. Our phone rang at 12:00 p.m.; it was Jennifer. Her mum had made other plans, she told me, and had dropped Jennifer off in Banstead High Street three hours early. Jennifer asked if I could walk down and get her. At that moment, I realised that all good plans of mice and men were in, fact, screwed. I told my mum, and she would not let me cancel with Jan at such short notice. I begged her, and she stood firm. I had told Jennifer that I was friends with another girl, and rightly so, she was very jealous. So, when I walked down to the high street and met Jennifer and told her that Jan was coming for lunch, the shit hit the fan.

We all sat around our dining table, which was laid out every Sunday with a nice tablecloth, placemats, and cutlery. My mum sat at the head of the table, and Jennifer and Jan sat next to each other, with me in front of them both. My two sisters were there, too. To say you could cut the atmosphere with a knife would be a vast understatement . . . I have never in all my life felt as uncomfortable as at that moment. We sat in stony silence with just polite small talk breaking through, and because I was sitting opposite them both, I could feel Jennifer's wrath burrow deeply into my soul. A few weeks prior to this, Jennifer had gifted me a small leather necklace with beads on it. I'd thought little of it, so I had given it to Jan as a token of my friendship. It was about five minutes into the most torturous meal I have ever sat through when I realised Jan was wearing the necklace! I died a thousand deaths during that meal. I never understood how my mum could be so cruel in not letting me cancel, but I thought she was teaching me a valuable lesson, and she did. Jennifer was a lovely girl, and I am glad I had never cheated on her, but soon after, I found out she'd cheated on me. She told me, and we sat, and both cried, and I left very upset.

What happened next is difficult for me to share. One of them is admitting that what would happen next had nothing to do with Jennifer cheating on me. It happens in everyday life, especially when young. It was because I had a lot of issues with trust, and I felt the need to be loved unconditionally. What happened was a culmination of the trauma from my past. After finishing with Jennifer, I went to a pub with some friends to drown my sorrows. I drank and took an entire bottle of hay fever tablets, hoping to overdose. The next day, I woke up; my overdose attempt had not worked. I was working at a golf club as a part-time dishwasher. My mum dropped me off for work and within a short time, I became quite unwell. On top of the dishwasher machine, there was a scrunched-up towel, and as I walked past, the towel turned into a white lion's head and roared at me. I was startled but continued making my way into the staff break room, which was full of staff. Then I blacked out. The staff realised something was wrong, and I remember being worried. I walked back into the main kitchen and into the chilled food storage room. The shelves were laden with various foods, like cheeses, meats, and delicacies. For no reason at all, I walked over to a tray of miniature apple pies, the same as you would buy in a supermarket. The tops of the pies had two small pastry leaves for decoration, and to my amazement, the leaves opened like mouths and talked to me. In the squeakiest voice you could imagine, a tray load of Mr. Kipling apple pies all began begging me not to eat them. 'Please do not eat us,' they pleaded. Their little mouths opened as they spoke and I didn't know what to think, but I reassured them I would not eat them. The next thing I knew, my mum turned up. She had been called in by the staff, who did not know what was happening to me.

We got home, and I walked upstairs to the bathroom. For some reason, I took a big bite out of a bar of soap. I could see a large bite with teeth marks in the bar, and as the foul taste hit me, I said to myself how disgusting the taste was and that it tasted like soap. I spat it out and walked halfway down the stairs. My mum was on the phone to the hospital, speaking to the psychiatric team in a panic with no idea what was happening. I sat on the stairs and saw my younger sister's white school socks next to me. To this day, I have no idea why, but I picked up one of the socks, shoved it in my mouth, and tried to chew off a piece. My mum saw what I was doing, and whilst still in conversation with the psych team, asked me why I was chewing my little sister's school sock. I apologised and told her, 'I thought it was a bar of soap.' That was the moment the hospital decided I needed an urgent admission. I think they gave my mum a time later on to take me down because we all still sat down to lunch. My mum had made beef stew, and as I was eating it I saw a bay leaf in my dinner, except I didn't see a bay leaf. I saw a slug moving across my dinner. Horrified, I yelled at my mum that there was a slug in my dinner. My sisters sat at the table, sniggering. Later that day, my mum took us down to Epsom Hospital, and I had a parched mouth. Like most mums, she kept all sorts of things in her handbag, so I asked her if she had a boiled sweet. She found a rather old Werther's Original and gave it to me. I took one look at it and said, 'I'm not eating that after you've pissed, shit, and farted on it.' I think that this is one of the funniest things I have ever said to anyone in my entire life, and every now and then, it pops up in the family conversation and we all giggle.

The next few days were a haze, but I remember my nan visited and I got up out of bed and lifted a huge hospital fire door off its hinges with ease and handed it to her, telling her it was for her. They had done blood tests and figured out that I had overdosed on my hay fever tablets. I was to be kept under close observation. I had different plans and even though I was on the first floor, I jumped out of the window, with no harm to my body, and decided to walk home. I had no idea where I was and ended up on the nearby Ashtead Common. As I wandered about, I bumped into three of my friends and we chatted briefly. I remember telling them I knew they were hallucinations, but could they give me directions home? After a very long time, I somehow made my way home. It was probably a good thirteen miles, and by this point, my mum and the hospital staff were looking for me. So, when I turned up, they were more than a bit relieved. I only remember one more thing during the whole episode, which lasted about a week. Every object around me had a green-and-red fuzzy line around it. It moved and frizzled like something out of a science fiction film, a bit like electricity. Everything I looked at had this, and I remember looking at my arm and was fascinated by this strange red-and-green energy pulsating around the outside.

Within a week, the effects wore off, and I was fine. I saw a psychiatrist who asked me if I regretted my overdose, and I told him yes, and they did no more tests. He told me that emotions are a lot stronger for teenagers and that, as I grew up, my emotions would settle down. In hindsight, I think he should have dug harder to find out why I was suicidal and offered me counselling or psychotherapy. It was a horrible experience, more so for my family and especially my poor mum who, as usual, would always be there for me no matter what throughout my life.

Chapter Seven
Trendle Mechanical Services

After they kicked me out of college for poor attendance, I found myself in our kitchen with my mum. Annoyed with me, she suggested I work for my grandfather and uncles who owned a large plumbing and construction company. We made a call to my uncle, and he offered me a labouring job. They gave me an address of a housing estate in Croydon and told me to be there before 8:00 a.m. and to dress in work clothes and steel-toe cap boots. I had no transport at the time, so I had to catch a few busses.

It was midwinter and at 6:20 a.m., I stood and waited at the bus stop, in the bitter dark and cold, shivering from head to toe. I am not even sure how I planned the route or found the address with no internet back then. At 8:00 a.m., I sat in a run-down squat of a house at a desk with the contracts manager, whom I addressed as 'sir'. The room was the site office for the foreman and filled with large blueprints, muddy boots, and various equipment. They laughed every time I called him 'sir', and the supervisor ribbed him at being spoken to politely and respectfully. Although respect is given on building sites, tradesmen are not known for formalities. I look back now at how kind he was to me.

I seemed to fit in well on-site. We worked very hard, but we had so much fun. I loved being around some of the other guys. It was like being at a stand-up comedy club if you worked with the right guys all day. There were some horrible bastards, too, though. A group of 'Chippies' disliked one guy, and, imagining he was earning more than them, they stole his tools. I found myself in a troublesome situation which even now I would struggle with. I overheard them, and they knew I had overheard them. Stealing a tradesperson's tools is as low as it gets. Without tools, you cannot work and earn money. The site was unhappy that it had happened, and I knew who had done it. Did I want to be labelled the 'grass' of the company and never be trusted, and very probably have the living shit kicked out of me? Or did I want to do the right and moral thing and let a man go back to work without spending a lot of money to replace his tools? The choice hurt me, but it was the right one: I said nothing. But I would always despise that gang and I never trusted them. Over the years, I saw a fair bit of theft – some minor copper pipes and fittings for private work were fair game, but when people stole boilers, big bundles of copper to sell, and the site's red diesel, it pissed me off, and although I said nothing . . . I knew.

After my first week at work, Friday evening, I received my little brown envelope. I did not open it until I got home. I called my mum into our kitchen and she watched me excitedly open it. Inside was a payslip and cash notes with coins. I can't remember for sure, but I think it was £112. My mum asked to see it. I handed it over with a big smile on my face. She counted it out and took £37, put it on the worktop, and said that was for my rent. I was furious with her; my blood boil and the rage build up inside of me. 'That is my hard-earned wages. You cannot do that!' I told her. She shut me down and told me I ate more than that a week, and that a third of my wages was to pay for my keep. I stormed upstairs with my £75, feeling unfairly treated. Now I look back and chuckle at how spoiled and entitled I was, and it taught me very early that no matter how little you give, pay your way in life. And if my kids ever moved in with me, even if I were wealthy, I would do the same to them, if only to teach them the same valuable lesson.

My social life in Banstead was particularly good. I had a lot of friends from college, and they drove, so we would visit pubs for a quiet pint. My favourite pub in the village was The Victoria. It was so welcoming and vibrant, and in all the years I drank in there, I never saw a single fight. I would spend most evenings in the pub with Joe and sometimes George. We began drinking there from the age of seventeen, and underage drinking was not frowned upon if you were sensible, which we were. Over time, I knew the regulars, who were always cheerful, and Friday and Saturday nights became the highlight of the week. The more people I got to know, the more I felt I belonged and became quite popular over the years. By the age of eighteen, there was a large crowd of us that would hang out and go to nightclubs and make day trips to the beach. It was a lovely, joyful time for me.

Chapter Eight
Sarah

My friends and I heard that ten miles away was a lively pub called The Stoneleigh Inn. It held a party night every Thursday night with a live DJ that played dance music but also held fun games, like people dressing up in black bin bags, and we started going every week. Life was working hard, partying hard, and it was a delicate balance at eighteen. One night at Stoneleigh Inn, I met a girl called Sarah. She was a year younger than me with blonde permed hair and was the spitting image of Top Gun's Kelly McGillis. She lived close in Tadworth and we were soon an item, spending a lot of our time together.

At seventeen, I had passed my motorcycle test and bought myself a brand-new motorbike, a Yamaha RD 350 YPVS, in black. We went everywhere on my bike, even visiting the Isle of White for a brief break. After eight months, Sarah finished school and started nurse training. They awarded her a place at Barts Hospital and she soon moved into her halls of residence. I visited twice a week, and although it was a ball ache to get there, I didn't mind. One fateful evening, she told me she was off work, so I paid her a surprise visit. I went to sign in the register only to be told she was out, and I saw it was with another guy who had signed in to see her. I felt heartbroken and betrayed. I sat in the reception hall for over an hour, sobbing my heart out. Student nurses walked past me, and they ignored me. At that moment, I realised people don't care, as not a single soul came over to ask what was up and maybe comfort me. And that hurt just as much. If I saw someone sobbing in the street, I wouldn't forgive myself if I did not offer comfort. I wandered the London streets searching for Sarah, which was of course ridiculous, until yet again, the despair welled deep inside of me. I bought a bottle of whisky and some paracetamol and drank. I had the foresight to call George and his girlfriend, Carly. They drove up to London and picked me up, no questions asked. I got over my heartbreak, but little did I know, it was another demon of mistrust for women I would later have to face.

I had been friends with Carly whilst I was at college and had introduced her to George, who was smitten with her.

She was an attractive girl with a bubbly personality, and we were quite close. George and Carly dated for maybe a year, and we spent a lot of time together as a group of friends. One evening, George and Carly had a big falling out, and he drove off in a frenzy. I found out she had told him she was in love with me and could not be with him. This sent me into a whirlwind of guilt and turmoil. I felt so awful for George that someone had broken his heart because of me and I tried so hard to be there for him. But it was too much for him to bear, and he shut me out of his life. It was a stupid thing for Carly to do; she should have made an excuse that would not have ruined my and George's friendship.

I felt a deep loss for many years. George was a hero of mine, someone I looked up to, and he was a pillar of strength for me. One example was when a group of us had been to a party. I was with Jennifer at that time, and there were about seven of us guys walking along a shopping walkway. A group of six thugs approached me and Jennifer, and it kicked off. I ushered her away, and George and one other friend came back to stand up to the thugs. Four of our other so-called mates walked off and watched us from one hundred metres away in safety and did nothing. There were six of them and three of us, but it was a good scrap and we did ourselves proud. We walked away, but word soon got around that the four who stood by and watched had lost an awful lot of respect, and we considered them cowards.

That was the George I loved – a kind and loyal friend. Carly and I remained friends for some time, and what had happened was never mentioned. Nothing ever happened between us, and even if it had, I think I would have pushed it away out of respect for George. Her friendship was more important to me as well.

Chapter Nine
Plumbing

By the time I reached eighteen, my labouring job at Trendles was becoming tedious, although I worked hard. My boss asked me one day if I would like to learn a trade and I jumped at this chance. They asked me which trade I fancied and, being a plumbing company, it was a simple choice. I spent six months with different plumbers to learn the ropes and spent one day at college studying for my City and Guild craft in plumbing. Depending on whom they paired me with, the work was more interesting and fun than my previous labouring job. There was a lot of travel involved, and by this time, I had passed my driving test and had a car, a lovely silver Ford Capri 2.0 Sport. Some jobs were miles away and would take me two and a half hours to get home from, which exhausted me.

My new position as an apprentice plumber varied between working on building sites and refurbishments on council estates in London, which I hated. Some flats were pigsties. I remember one which was full of about seven medical students. The place stank of body odour and was vile, with leftover food and dirty plates strewn all over the place. One day, we had to fit a radiator on a wall in one of the three bedrooms and a student was asleep in a bed by the wall. We asked him to move, and he ignored us, so we had to pick up the bed with him in it and drill through a concrete wall . . . which was loud. He just turned over and went back to sleep. I remember feeling complete contempt for them, living like pigs.

Life on-site was never dull. Each trade sat in a shipping container that housed our supplies and tools. All we had was a kettle and a lunch box of sandwiches. We started at 8:00 a.m. and we finished at 4:00 or 5:00 p.m. depending on the time of year. Sometimes we played cards at lunch, or read the paper, or just talked shit. There were the usual high jinks, such as my foreman trying to send me out for elbow grease, but I never fell for any of them. Despite my grandad being the owner of the company, and my uncles, the directors, I was shown no nepotism at all; in fact, quite the opposite: I was put with the hardest bastards in the company, and in hindsight, I know it was to toughen me up and earn respect. When I saw my family in the office, I always addressed them like you would a boss, using 'sir'.

One day, just before my lunch break, I decided it would be hilarious to nail my plumbing foreman's lunch box to the workbench and glue the lid shut with mastic. He tried to open it and couldn't, and I burst out laughing – that is, until he picked up an iron gas pipe and chased me around the site for twenty minutes , screaming abuse at me. I soon learnt not to fuck with the hard bastards. There were other funny incidents, such as the time an electrician called me from a different room. As I grabbed the handle of the door, I had a huge painful shock. He had put his electrical mega tester on the handle on the other side and it gave me a good belt. I got him back with a copper blowpipe. I used a three-foot piece of fifteen-millimetre copper pipe and placed a small piece of plumber's mait, took aim, and blew. Even at twenty feet away, if that hit you in the neck, you would know about it. I spent a many a time hiding in upstairs windows with a putty gun and would only shoot electricians, who were our arch-rivals.

I would duck down, and they never knew what happened; you would just hear them scream. A teaspoon left in boiling tea while it brewed was occasionally picked up and put against our necks. Man, that hurt.

Chapter Ten
Jan

My social life was thriving during this time, and I spent most nights down at my local pub, The Vic in Banstead, and in nightclubs such as The Blue Orchid in Croydon on weekends. One night, I bumped into Jan at a local club. We had not seen each other in years, and she invited me back to hers. Nothing happened; we just chatted, and I slept on the sofa. The next morning, the house was empty, and we spent the whole Sunday as if we were starring in a porno movie. Jan was a pretty, buxom girl with lovely long brunette hair and she dressed well. She had a great sense of humour, very silly just like mine, so we had a lot of fun. Jan was also very fiery, as was I, and when we rowed, which was often, it was nasty.

Before Jan and I became an item, two of my friends and I had booked an 18-30s holiday to Magaluf in Majorca. I think Jan and I had been together maybe three months, and I had every intention of being faithful, but one of those 'funny stories' of mine happened on the second night. The first day my friends arrived at The Samos Hotel, we bumped into two girls staying a few rooms down. One girl was smoking hot, and the other, not so much. On our second night, we were quite tired and sitting in our room chatting when the girls knocked on our door and invited us to their room. We obliged and, even though I was only wearing my boxer shorts, nobody cared. As we sat chatting, laughing, and drinking vodka, I lay on the beds next to the hot one. Her friend and my two friends were sitting on the other bed, which was connected. I had a little feel and pulled the sheet over us, and before I knew it, we were shagging on our sides in front of the others. The hilarious thing was that you could not mistake what we were doing three feet away from my friends, but I kept chatting to them like nothing was happening. 'So what time are we hitting the beach tomorrow, guys?' I asked as I was pounding away. As the evening progressed, one of my mates copped off with the other one and we slept over. From what I can gather, she was on a mission to get a different guy every night, and she did. I got back from my holiday, and Jan and my mum collected me from the airport. When we got home, I told her what had happened and told her I was sorry, but if she could forgive me, I would never cheat again. She told me she had stayed at some friend's house and a similar thing had happened but reckoned she only got her boobs out . . . yeah, right. Funny thing is, every time we rowed, she would throw my infidelity at me.

I have a lot of amazing memories of my time with Jan. We would go out on a Friday night down to The Vic, get drunk, go back to mine, and cram into my single bed. Every Saturday morning was spent in bed, watching Saturday Morning Live with Phillip Schofield and Gordon the Gopher. We went out most Saturday afternoons, shopping at either Sutton or Epsom. We would mooch around the shops and end up having McDonald's. I loved nothing more than browsing around WH Smith, looking at my favourite books, or checking out all the cool stuff in The Gadget Shop. One afternoon, whilst we were in Epsom, a stranger approached me in the Ashley Centre and gave me a big smile, saying to me, 'You're Darren Smith, aren't you?'

'Yes,' I replied. 'Who are you?' I asked her.

She continued with, 'You live at 85 Brighton Road, Banstead, Surrey, SM6 8QX, don't you?'

It took me aback and I looked at Jan.

'Who are you?' I asked the stranger.

She was middle-aged, with shoulder-length hair and brown eyes. I had no idea who she was. She then told me my date of birth, grinned, and walked off. What had just happened? Who was she?

I could not chase after her, and we did not have mobile phones, so I could not get her picture to show around. This encounter mystified me for years.

Another one of my 'funny stories': One evening, Jan and I went for a drive to a local beauty spot. The car park was empty, so we got down to the business, and I spied a car pulling up some way over yonder with its lights on. It worried me that it could be the police or perverts, so I sped up, finished, and pulled up my trousers. We drove home, and it was late.

Jan was sitting in my room, and I went into the bathroom and sat on the toilet, quite tired. As I urinated, I felt this strange feeling on my dick, and the only way I can describe it was like a cow being milked. I looked down, and to my amazement realised that in my haste to pull up my trousers in the car park, I had not taken off the condom. The condom was still on me, half-filled with pee and wobbling all over the place, tugging on my dick. I burst out laughing and called Jan in to look.

Word soon got out about my funny stories, and I'm not sure what people my age thought about me. Another evening, Jan and I were in a rather compromising situation in my bedroom. I was pretty much left alone when I was in the bedroom, and my mum was downstairs watching TV. Whilst we were enjoying our sexy time, we heard a brief knock on my door, and without time to yell out, 'Not at the moment!', the door opened and my mother walked straight in. She stood shocked as she saw us in the 69 position and shouted, 'Jesus Christ, it's like a Chinese brothel in here!' and stormed out. I don't think I looked at my mum for a week afterwards, and I have never enjoyed a blow job since. Jan was very promiscuous behind my back, but I was way too naïve to realise this at the time. She once got genital warts and then gave them to me . . . I should have known, but she had told me she had a wart on her hand and it had spread.

My best mate at the time was a guy named Neil. He worked in the civil service and, although quiet, was great fun and intelligent. We began weight training at a local spit-and-sawdust gym in Sutton called The Workhouse. We trained three times a week, and if I'm honest, we looked bloody good. We were slim and muscular. After the gym, we would head down to a different pub each time, taking it in turns to drive. There were so many lovely pubs in Surrey, and we would just pick one afterwards. Often, when we got down to The Vic, there would be about fifteen of us sitting around having fun and drinking. The pub was next to a Waitrose supermarket and there were shopping trolleys everywhere. Many times, I went out to my car to find a Waitrose shopping trolley on the roof of my car. It became a standing joke that you never left the pub last, and we gave as good as we got.

Work was also going well, and I finally finished my fourth year at college and received my City and Guilds advanced craft in plumbing. I spent hours doing my coursework and drawing very technical drawings in colour along with writing long essays, and when I finished, my lecturers asked me if they could keep them to show future students what they could do. I was honoured, but I wish I had kept them as a reminder of how studious I was.

My grandad passed away when I was about nineteen years old, and it hit me quite hard. He was a lovely, kind man with a great sense of humour. He was old-school and was the typical man of the house who expected tea at 3:30 p.m. in a bone china teacup with a biscuit, with dinner ready on the table each evening. But my lovely nan never went without, and she was the most amazing, loving woman. My grandad passed away at a football match watching his favourite team, Crystal Palace, with my uncle. He had a scotch in one hand and a big fat cigar in the other, and it was instant. I don't think he could have wished for a better way to go.

My three uncles ran TMS Ltd, but the cracks showed between them and soon there was a power struggle. There was a big split, and one uncle left, taking half the staff and work and setting up on his own. My other uncle struggled and was left with the less profitable side of the work – new site work – and sadly, the firm went under. There was a huge rift within the family following this, and it all got ugly and Trendles went into bankruptcy. I tried to stay out of it, and I was lucky enough to find work with an industrial plumbing and pipefitting company called AG Manly in Wandsworth. The work was unique, as it was on an industrial scale and I thought it would broaden my skill set. It involved fitting long lengths of six-inch cast iron 'Timesaver' drainage hanging from 'spits' in the concrete ceilings of car parks. It was very, very hard work and was done underground with lamp lights to see. I was with AG Manly for maybe two years before the recession hit hard and we were all laid off.

I was a fully qualified advanced plumber and an associate with the Institute of Plumbing, which showed I was experienced enough to supervise plumbers on-site. After my course finished, I won two awards, of which I was very proud. I won my company's student achievement award and the Institute of Plumbers award for achievement made during my studies. I have kept all of my certificates collected over the years, and from time to time I look through them fondly. After being laid off in 1992 because of the terrible recession, finding work within the industry was impossible. I began thinking about which direction I wanted my life to go, and I was very keen to continue my studies, so I enquired about studying full-time for an HND in mechanical services at the same college, NESCOT. The tutors turned me down for the course. They thought a lowly plumber would not cut the grade. I was quite cross, as I was more than capable of studying hard. I was bright and hardworking. They say every time a door closes, a new one opens. And that happened in the form of a foundation degree course in NESCOT. The course was to prepare mature students for a degree and was broadly based within construction. I called the course leader, a lovely man called Gary, and he explained NESCOT was one of many satellite colleges running the course, and that it led onto South Bank University once completed.

Chapter Eleven
Foundation Degree

I headed down for a formal interview with South Bank University with a very dull, stiff lecturer who tested my basic arithmetic knowledge, and I came up woefully short. My second interview was at NESCOT with Gary, the course lead, and it went very well and we got on. He explained all the course modules, projects, and exams and what I could expect. I explained to him that I had passed my Advanced City and Guilds with merits and distinctions, and being a NESCOT student stood me in good stead. I was accepted a couple of days later via a phone call from Gary, and I was so excited to tell my mum. I remember feeling like I was back on track and my mum was so proud. Heading to university was a rare thing in the nineties and nobody in our family had been before.

There were about eighteen people in my class, all guys about my age and the eldest, maybe thirty-five. The course was full-time nine to five every day, although we got breaks to research projects and for library study. As the course began in September 1993, I had to apply for a grant to live on, which was a meagre £690 for each six-month term. I decided I had to find part-time work if I stood any chance of supporting myself and paying something towards rent. I began looking for work and was lucky to find evening and Saturday work at a local convenience store called

Dayton's on Banstead High Street. Before long, I was working three or four nights a week and Saturdays. The work was varied and the great camaraderie, infectious. The manager was a guy my age named Mike; he was the most charismatic and hardworking guy I had ever met, and he taught me so much. He and his deputy manager, Carl, lived above a shop in the high street, and when the shift finished, we would pop the shop keys in his letterbox. Mike took me under his wing and we got on well – we were both very ambitious, striving for perfection and recognition.

Jan and I always had a rocky relationship, and we argued a lot. According to my sisters, I would wind her up like a mouse and let her go. When we rowed, we screamed, and it was unhealthy, but within a couple of days, we would make up. Jan was a very ambitious girl who worked for a huge insurance company and was a team leader of six, which for her age was a respectable career progression. Jan and I mixed a little with the Dayton's lot. I worked with a young guy called Jeff; he was seventeen, geeky, religious, and very academic. I liked him, so on Friday night, during work, I asked him if he wanted to come next door to The Vic for a pint with us. Jan and I got there first, grabbed a table and a drink, and Jeff walked in fifteen minutes later. I smiled at him and asked him what he wanted. Sheepishly he said, 'Well, you invited me.' Jan and I wet ourselves laughing, as when I'd asked him what he wanted, it had meant what he would like to drink. I playfully corrected him and bought him a pint.

My youngest sister, Melanie, had been dating a guy called Albert for a year. I got on well with him and considered him a good friend. He was an engineer for a large aircraft company, working on jumbo jets; he worked hard and earned very good money. The four of us spent a lot of time together, even going to Spetses, one of the Greek islands, for a holiday. Halfway through my foundation year, Jan went out one Friday night with my sister and Albert. They visited one of Albert's old friends and they all ended up staying over. I found out the next day that Jan had slept with the guy and that finished us. My demon popped his head up once more and I just could not trust women.

I found myself in uncharted waters, single and with no responsibilities apart from college and a part-time job. So, I did what any other twenty-three-year-old guy would do: I threw myself into party mode. My foundation degree year was coming to its end in 1993, and I had excelled in all subjects, except maths. I was very disappointed that I had not passed and spoke to my tutor, Gary, who offered to home tutor me once a week. That summer, Gary taught me every week for three months. He lived a good fifty minutes away and he was very kind to me. I cannot remember, but I hope I paid him for his time. I sat my maths exam later in September 1993 and aced it, thanks to Gary. At the end of my foundation degree year, they gave me two awards. One was from NESCOT College for my achievement. I attended a ceremony, which I was proud of, and featured in a NESCOT College newsletter promoting the course. And they awarded me the Baroness Perry Award for the student who had made the biggest improvement on my course within all satellite colleges. My tutor and course lead, Gary, put me forward with a powerful endorsement. I attended a ceremony at South Bank University and was given a certificate and £1,000. I felt very honoured and just wanted my mum to feel that I had turned a new leaf and be proud of me.

Over the summer of 1993, I worked full-time at Dayton's whilst waiting to start at South Bank University in September. Most of the staff were older teens, a few older ladies, and a couple of us guys in our early twenties. I have so many fond memories of working with the younger staff. In our small kitchen area, we had a kettle and a sandwich toastie maker. Every Saturday, we would try to outdo one another with the most outlandish toasties. I think my baked bean, cheese, and mayo toastie did well. The work was mundane, but we were all hard workers and took pride in everything we did. The shop was immaculate every night when we locked up. And I always polished the floor like a pin with one of those funny machines that spun around. It almost became a competition – who could lock up with the cleanest store. All the tins and bottles 'faced up' so precisely and anally retentively, it made me smile inside. I threw myself into having fun and getting drunk, having a laugh whenever I could. I was popular, slim, handsome, and fun to be around. As time went by, I got wilder in my behaviour. The flat where Mike and Carl lived was filled most evenings with local friends who would sit around and smoke hash. We would regularly smoke it to the point where we passed out. This became a regular occurrence, and at midnight after a session, I would take the stoned walk of shame home and sneak in, trying to not wake anyone.

My younger sister, Melanie, was bored with Albert. She dumped him and we found ourselves in the same situation. And whilst Albert smoked a lot of hash, he didn't mix in the same circles as the Dayton's lot. I became good friends with a guy called Philip who was a few years younger than me and studying at university. He worked at Dayton's when he was on university break and we got on well. He was intelligent, very kind-hearted, and caring. His sister, Joy, also worked at Dayton's and was a friendly girl, slightly younger. One day, it was found out she had damaged a packet of crisps to write them off. Writing off an item means making a note of the item and cost, and it is then meant to be thrown away. Unfortunately, she damaged the packet and wrote the crisps off to eat them. It appalled me when they sacked her for this minor indiscretion and made an example of her.

I met a girl called Rebecca at a local party; she had a figure to die for, long wavy white-blonde hair, and was cute. We got on well and saw each other for a little while, but I broke it off a couple of months in, as I didn't feel as keen as she did. She slept with a couple of my friends, including Albert, out of revenge. I wasn't jealous, but it pissed me off that a friend like Albert would sleep with my ex. I spoke to him about it, but he didn't get it, which annoyed me even more.

Our meeting point from Dayton's was next door, The Victoria in Banstead High Street, which had been my favourite haunt for years. There were maybe twenty of us who hung out and all got on well together. One night at the bar when I was ordering a drink, a young girl I knew called Winnie tapped me on the shoulder. She was eighteen years old and studying for A levels. I turned and smiled at her, asking what she wanted, and she shocked me to the core when she asked me outright if she could give me a blow job. I declined, but my friend Carl, with his boyish looks, had heard what she had asked and told her he would accept her offer. From that moment on, they were an item, and she moved in. Last I heard, they are still together. I look back now and wonder how he could have a long-term relationship with a girl who had offered his mate a blow job and he was second choice. The tone during that year seemed like a long party filled with drugs, sex, and studying.

During my time at Dayton's, I had a major crush on a girl there called Charlotte. She had a long-time boyfriend, but that did not stop me from flirting with her. She never wavered from her boyfriend, but in hindsight, I was a complete bastard to him and her. I heard they settled down, married, and had children. I feel a lot of remorse for my behaviour, but I was out of control.

Chapter Twelve
Sue

During the late summer of 1993, I pulled up outside the pub on one of my motorbikes, a ratty Yamaha RD 400. There were lots of friends sitting outside on the patio. I chatted with a few of them, and a young girl, whom I would later get to know, named Sue came over, asking questions and flirting. She seemed quite young, and whilst very attractive, I brushed her off as a pest. Within a couple of months, I bumped into her at Mike's flat where there must have been about ten people sitting around getting stoned. It surprised me to see her, and she seemed to have grown overnight from an annoying teenager into a beautiful young woman. We chatted that evening and from that moment, I seemed to bump into her everywhere I went. As she had blossomed, the whole of the pub and half of Banstead had fallen for her.

Occasionally, a few of us from Banstead went into nearby Sutton, the nearest large shopping town, to a dive of a pub that had a big disco. It was a very rough pub and was known for its patrons getting paralytic and fighting. One night after drinking a sizable amount of 20/20 Mad Dog, it kicked off outside, and I squared up to two guys. I took off my T-shirt off and went into full yob mode. I don't even know what the fight was about, but there were maybe thirty people outside kicking off. Thankfully, nothing happened, but I am ashamed of the person I was back then. Another evening, a vast group ended up at the pub, and we bumped into the Banstead postmen. They were a good bunch of about twelve guys who hung out together and just enjoyed a drink. After the night ended, everyone went for a curry. We took over the restaurant with maybe twenty-two of us. I sat with Mike, Carl, and Winnie, and we ordered our meal. Sitting back afterwards, we were chatting when I realised Mike had disappeared. I thought it odd, as he had been gone for some time, so I checked the toilets in case he had passed out drunk. He was nowhere to be seen, so I went back to the others and we realised he had walked out and not paid, and that we would have to pick up the tab. Carl told me he wasn't paying and was thinking about leaving, too. I became cross that they could do such a thing and expect me to pay for all of them, so I did something I still very much regret. I walked over to a few postmen who were sitting by the front door and began chatting to them. Then, when the server's back was turned, I grabbed the door hard and ran out. I have never run so hard in all my life, and in my mind's eye, I felt there were five Indian men chasing me with meat cleavers. The next day, I met up with Carl and asked him what had happened, and he told me he and Winnie walked to the door where they were met by a server. They thanked him for a lovely meal and walked out without paying, too.

Albert, my sister's ex, moved into his nan's bungalow since she had recently passed, and whilst it was on the market, his father felt it wise to keep it occupied. Albert invited me to move in. Before long, there were a couple of parties and Albert began dating Joy, the girl from Dayton's, and they made a nice couple. At this point, Sue and I had become good friends, and I began inviting her back to the bungalow. It was not long after that that Sue and I became very much a couple. We kept it hushed up until one Friday night in a different local pub filled with friends, I grabbed her in my arms and kissed her passionately. Our friends gasped in shock, and then they all cheered and laughed. Sue had experimented, as some teenagers do, with some harder drugs such as LSD, mushrooms, speed, and ecstasy. She was into the rave scene, and one evening down at a different pub, she showed me a flyer for a huge rave called World Dance in Lydd Airport on the coast. They advertised a funfair, two different rooms and a host of famous underground DJs. I got sucked in and began listening to rave music and thought about trying ecstasy.

I worked Christmas Eve at Dayton's in 1993, but at 10:00 p.m., we raced next door to The Vic, who had their annual disco in full swing. I tried some speed (amphetamine) and foolishly bought two 'wraps' at £10 a wrap. Most first-time users would try half a wrap, but I decided I knew better. They came wrapped up in a piece of Rizla paper and I swallowed them. Within thirty minutes, I came up and was buzzing off my face. On amphetamines, you feel so full of energy to the point that you cannot stay still and just want to dance, and it also makes you feel an intense euphoria. I made my way home, and Christmas was spent at my nan's in Tadworth. She had a lovely five-bedroom new build, and I felt so at home there. Because of the effects of the two wraps of speed, I was still off my face and spent at least three days in bed, unable to sleep and on a major comedown. I told my family I had fallen ill with something and they left me to it. I now understand why they call taking amphetamines 'running with the devil', as I lay there awake for seventy-two hours, exhausted, depressed, confused, shaking, and shivering.

In September 1993, I had begun my first-year degree in construction management (con man for short) at South Bank University. I did not feel at home at the college at all; it was very dreary, cold, and unwelcoming. They held some classes in the main auditorium and some in smaller classrooms. Most of the lessons were generic built environment classes that hosted all construction students, such as architectural and surveying degrees. I found the classes like economics and statistics held no relevance to construction. We also had a science class that was difficult, and I felt like I was struggling. Travelling to uni every day was a pain, so I shared a lift with a classmate, Andrew. To say I found Andrew annoying is an understatement. He had been in my previous year at NESCOT and was the class fool, and he just got under my skin. But he was kind enough to give me lifts, so I shouldn't backbite him.

Looking back now, I realise that my mental health was in a downward spiral. I was not only burning the candle at both ends with study and part-time work; I was burning it in the middle by socialising with Sue and getting stoned every night. Andrew and his friends started hanging out at our local pubs and were also into the rave scene, and we all got sucked in further. My friend Carl at Dayton's pulled me to one side at one point and told me not to mess around with hard drugs. He told me not to do the ecstasy I was planning on taking, going on to tell me a story about a guy who took LSD and never came down. He told me that the guy spent the rest of his life constantly hallucinating; I wish I had listened to Carl.

Chapter Thirteen
Ecstasy

One night, my good friend from Dayton's, Philip, and I hit a rave club in Islington in London. John and Andrew from college and a friend of Andrew's came too. Philip and I bought an ecstasy tablet from Charlotte's boyfriend. As we queued to get into Paradise, Philip and I took the ecstasy tablet. It was called a 'white dove' because embossed onto the tablet was a picture of a dove. These tablets were strong and, it being our first time, we were cautious, so Philip took half, and I took a whole one. We got into the club and it was really dingy with very dark red walls. The music was so loud, you could barely hear anything. The music was deep jungle music, which I didn't like. It felt very sinister. Philip and I sat down on one of the long-padded seats and waited for the ecstasy to work, but it did not. After an hour of sitting, I told Philip I was going to see if I could buy another one. I caught some random bloke's eye, so I approached him. He handed over a white dove and I handed him £15. As I walked back to Philip, I swallowed the pill without hesitation. Little did I know that that minor act of putting a tablet in my mouth would have such an enormous impact on the rest of my life.

Within twenty minutes, the ecstasy hit me hard. I have never felt so awful and wretched. I began hallucinating with my hands. It is called 'tracking', and when I moved my hands in front of me, they left trails behind. It was odd. The mood in the club took a dark dive and became almost demonic. I began 'rushing' up my back. The only way I can describe it is like a massive orgasm starting at the base of my spine, shooting up to my neck. I felt embarrassed by this, as it felt like a tremendous orgasm every ten seconds. I was worried, so my friends came over and I told them what was happening. I cannot remember much apart from them taking me out to the area in reception and buying me a pint of orange juice. Vitamin C makes you vomit when you take ecstasy and brings you down.

I sat down against a wall, next to what looked like an old professor. He could not have looked more out of place if he had tried. He had salt-and-pepper hair and he was propped up against the wall reading a book. I puked on the floor and no one took any notice. I am shocked now that no staff came over to see if I was okay, as I was not. Eventually, we went back to our seats, and Andrew and his friend went off to dance to the awful music. After a while, I realised I recognised someone, a face I had not seen in a long time. It was an old school friend, Neil, with his girlfriend, a nurse called Sarah. We chatted and caught up a little, but it was difficult because I was off my face and had become hypervigilant. Hypervigilance is a term used in mental health circles for those suffering from serious trauma. It heightened all of my senses beyond belief as the drug coursed through my body. I saw things in minute detail. The real problem was about to happen as I sat there. I saw a guy with what looked like a prosthetic ear. As I studied him and he moved in the dazzling lights, I saw it was not a prosthetic ear but a covert earpiece that you see in spy movies – it looked like see-through plastic moulded around the ear. I became very frightened that the police were at the club, and we had heard a poor young girl had overdosed on ecstasy in the club the week before, so it would make sense for them to be there. I looked around and saw other young people in their twenties with the same earpieces, and I became overcome with fear and paranoia brought on by the ecstasy. In my state of hypervigilance, I watched them as they worked as a team and I became aware they were watching me . . . and then shit got real.

My friends had left the club and by choice, I stayed, although I do not know why. At about five a.m., I left and, still off my face, got the tube to Trafalgar Square. Sitting in front of me on the tube were two guys from the club. I could see their earpieces, and I felt so frightened, like I had gotten caught up in a horror movie and couldn't get out. Why follow me? What had I done? What was happening? I felt so paranoid and extremely ill. Somehow, I got to the bus stop in Trafalgar Square and stood against the concrete bus timetable post looking for my bus time. As I looked at it, an attractive tall girl with long curly blonde hair stood and pretended to look at the other side of the timetable. I pretended to ignore her, but I recognised her from Paradise and she peeked around a few times at me. She was looking into my face. I saw her earpiece just like the others, which just compounded my fears even more. I was being followed and watched. I eventually got home confused and paranoid and went to bed in sheer dread. From that moment onwards, I was paranoid on two counts: one, because of the terrible trip I had had on ecstasy; and two, because I had been followed and watched. It was a good recipe for psychosis.

In hindsight, I should have spoken to my mum about what had happened, but I did not want her to know I had been smoking cannabis or messing around with class A drugs. I went to college and spoke to a few of the guys, and John told me that there had been a guy with a prosthetic ear but nothing else, but I knew he was trying to comfort me. As time went on, I was still at university, working part-time, living with Albert in Coulsdon, and dating Sue. Albert was spending more time with his new girlfriend, Joy, and she had a calming influence on him, so they stayed in more. But I carried on partying.

Sue and Andrew were really stoked about World Dance at Lydd Airport. We bought our tickets and paid for the coach trip, and before long, we were travelling down to the coast. It was a chilly night, and I was wearing jeans, a T- shirt, and a denim jacket. I was told not to dress too warm, as we would dance all night and ecstasy makes you hot as hell, which is why you see ravers drinking a lot of water. It is also easy to get dehydrated and that can be fatal. We queued to get in, and some random teenager from the coach latched onto us. I thought it was kind of strange, a kid going to a rave on his own, but we let him tag along. Andrew and his mates turned up, and he gave me my pill, which he had concealed in his cheek in tinfoil. I went off to find a huge row of Portaloos, as I was dying for the toilet. Whilst I was walking back to the enormous warehouse, I had an unusual encounter: A large security guard came charging towards me, glaring right at me like he was going for me, and I shat myself. Just as he was about to barge into me, he veered around me, and that was the moment I felt like I was being 'gaslighted'.

Gaslighting is the name of a film where a husband turns his wife psychotic by slowly turning down the gaslights in their Victorian home every week. She would complain it was getting darker and he would berate her and call her mad. In the end, he made her mad. The incident with the security guard frightened me, and whilst now I can think it might have been quite innocent, at the time, it felt very real, as if someone were messing with my head.

I popped the ecstasy tablet in my water bottle, and within half an hour, it kicked in. I remember it rushing up my spine, and I felt embarrassed as the orgasmic feeling repeated over and over. I tried to dance but didn't enjoy it, so after a while, I went for a walk around the warehouse. The laser and light show was amazing, with professional dancers on stages and podiums. The DJs were changed every hour with massive applause, as we knew them all. The music was old-school rave mixed up with drum and bass.

I bumped into the lone teenager and he asked if he could have some water. I gave him a gulp, but then remembered I had put my ecstasy in it and told him afterwards. He looked shocked, which surprised me, as he had told us he had dropped some before and if there was any left, it was probably very dissolved. I made my way up to the dancers when a pretty girl grabbed my water, held the bottle up to the light, and took a swig. I felt a pang for the kid, realising there probably had still been ecstasy in there, and hoped he hadn't got any more.

I went back to the group and told Sue I felt ill again and asked if we could go sit down somewhere safe and get warm. She took me to a Red Cross marquee that was serving hot tea and had a tarpaulin laid out on the ground. I queued to get a cup and froze when I realised my money was gone. I only had a tenner, and I'd either dropped it or had been pickpocketed. Sue had no cash, so we sat on the floor and she held me close to her to warm me up. I don't know why we didn't beg for a cup or ask for medical care; I think I was too embarrassed and wanted to ride it out. Sue looked after me, reassuring me my paranoia was going to go and I would be fine. We got home and smoked a joint, which helps with the comedown of ecstasy, then spent the day in bed.

That night, our group of friends met at the pub and we spoke about the event, but I cannot recall saying much.

Chapter Fourteen
It Began

One night in the bungalow, I was smoking cannabis, and I heard a male voice from outside the large window say, 'You bastard.' I went into paranoid mode again and thought that the drug squad was keeping tabs on me by watching from the back garden through our curtainless open windows at night. From that moment onwards, I slid into madness. The next day, I was afraid I was being bugged, so I ripped up the carpets in my little orange Mini looking for bugs. I found a large round Casio battery and was convinced it was a listening device. I went inside and checked all the old phone cabling, looking for devices, but I wouldn't even have known what a bugging device looked like even if I'd found one.

In a panic, I found the Yellow Pages and looked up private detectives, finding one who dealt with surveillance on cheating husbands and wives. I asked him if he knew if this battery was a bug, and he told me he did not think so and asked me if I was into any deep shit. I told him no but that I had been mucking around with drugs. He told me that the police would just kick my doors in if they were interested in me. I'm sure he knew I was unwell from what I had been saying and was trying to ease my fear, but it didn't work. My housemate, Albert, came in and I told him what had happened and he was concerned, and I remember him being confused about what I seemed to be going through.

That week was hell for me as my paranoid delusions grew and psychosis took hold. I went in to work and they had just installed a new computer to keep the data and records of customers' daily papers. I don't know why, but I scanned through the list looking at which customers had which paper and classifying them as left- or right-wing. My vision failed and everything seemed foggy, like I was in a smoky room, and I got frightened and felt out of control. Later that night, two of my young colleagues came in to see me and told me that there was a serious problem with theft that they knew about. Apparently, one guy I had asked to be promoted to supervisor had been unlocking the cigarette steel cage and swiping phone cards, stamps, and bundles of cartons of cigarettes. I was told it had been going on for a while and they wanted to report it. The guy who was doing it, Alex, had been a semi-drug friend, and I found myself in a difficult situation. On the one hand, he was a mate, but on the other, I had got him a promotion and he was stealing from the company that paid us and had therefore let me down, too. I told them to leave it to me, and I called the area manager. He camped out overnight in the car park and saw Alex put black bin liners in the industrial bins that evening on his shift. Later that night, Alex went back to the bins and took the black sacks with the stolen stuff hidden inside the bin liners. The area manager caught him red-handed, he was questioned, and as far as I'm aware, they let him go without prosecution.

I should have felt awful for dobbing him in, but I was psychotic, and my brain was confused and foggy. My vision was all over the place, and I was paranoid about everything and everyone. Every time I saw a car, I would check the number plate to see if I had seen it before. They installed something on the ceiling in the stockroom. Now and then it clicked and made me paranoid that it was a camera filming me. That evening, a teenager who worked there came up to me and said, 'It's probably a camera.' I shat myself, thinking he was in on something, as it was common knowledge his father was a police officer. I am sure it was a camera because of all the thieving that had been going on, but it felt like he had gaslighted me into becoming more unwell by saying that to me.

A day or so later, I moved back home to my mum's and gave up university. Sue stayed by my side and we spent a lot of time together trying to get through whatever it was I was experiencing. I would not talk about my experiences to anyone and pretended to be fine. I was too frightened to discuss it. One morning, I woke up and headed downstairs to the kitchen to make some coffee and popped on the little portable TV which was on the worktop. The programme was about finding God and becoming a born-again Christian. It hit me right in the face. I knew God was in my life; I just knew. I felt elated and complete, and as I looked out of our kitchen window, I saw a huge blossom of purple solanum flowers growing up against our wall on the patio. For some reason, seeing the purple flowers was a sign from God that He was with me, and this was His message. I walked down to Banstead and bumped into Joe, my geeky friend from Dayton's. Joe was very religious, and I felt it safe to tell him I had found God and could see it in every purple flower around me. He looked at me oddly and disbelievingly. This shocked me, as I knew he was a kid of deep faith. It felt like he thought I was not good enough to find faith. Soon after, Sue and I drove up to Lower Kingwood, which was not far. We went for a lovely walk and I looked up at the sky and prophesied. I picked out the two brightest stars in the sky and told her that these stars were moving closer together, and that when they met, all that would be left would be me and her in the garden of Eden.

It was soon my birthday, and Sue bought me an enormous bouquet of purple flowers and a balloon hanging outside. For the first time in ages, I felt half well. Sue stayed over a lot, and we dossed about most of the time, spending the rest of the time having wild sex. One night, I saw shadows on the walls and swore I saw one having sex with Sue whilst she slept. Again, I felt like I was trapped in a horror movie, and I shook with fear. I got up and went into my old small bedroom. I could hear the demons. I sat on the bed and sobbed and said to them, 'Do anything to me, but please do not harm Sue.' They agreed to this, it seemed.

Another night, we began having sex and she freaked out, telling me my eyes were glowing green. That night I could not sleep and was a mess, and I decided to take my life. I was tormented and in so much anguish, I was crying silently, so I ran a cold bath, lay down, fully submerged myself, and breathed in a lungful of water, hoping to drown myself. My body reacted, and I bolted upright and choked, coughed, and spluttered. I got dressed and went out for a cigarette. As I stood by our back door next to a wooden fence dividing our neighbours' property and ours, I was very distressed, panicking and crying, when I heard the hissing of gas. I could not explain the noise but felt calm. This would not be the last night I heard gas. Another time, I was sitting on the toilet and I could hear gas. I soon decided the gas was poisoning me. I became very paranoid, and I would have pulled up the floorboards had I not been stopped by Sue.

Chapter Fifteen
Dad's House

Sometime after this, Sue and I drove up to see my nan and bumped into her neighbour, a lovely older spinster with a very cute standard schnauzer called Ziggy. We asked her if we could take Ziggy for a walk, and she agreed. We drove with Ziggy, sixty miles away, to my dad's in Buckinghamshire. My dad was pleased to see us but a bit bewildered by the fact that we had kidnapped a dog from a little old lady from Surrey, and so he called my mum. My family turned up the next day, furious and confused as to why we would do such a thing.

By this time, Sue and I were both unwell, and I don't think it registered. The week we were at my dad's is a blur to me. We did strange things like drive up to churches, and one time I told a vicar off because his graveyard was very overgrown and needed care. I remember feeling like I was an emissary from God, showing my displeasure. I also drove around a lot doing good deeds, like picking up trash or helping people who were broken down on the side of the road. One night in my dad's lounge, I gave Sue a back massage, and she told me she had terrible asthma. I could see on her skin the outline of her lungs in black. I was convinced she had cancer and so, as I massaged her, I thought I was healing her. Afterwards, the black lung marks disappeared. The next day she had a terrible asthma attack, and I rushed her to Wycombe A&E. A poorly old man asked me what she was in for, and I told him lung cancer. Unsure what to say, he told me, 'And I thought I had problems.'

One night I could not sleep, so I decided to go for a drive, and in my mind, I was going to look for the devil and the gates of hell. I went out to my car, a beaten-up old orange Mini, and on the roof was a white plastic toy hobby horse. I had no idea what it meant, but in my madness, I found it significant, so I put it on the back seat and drove to a little town on the Thames called Marlow. It had been a lovely place we came to as kids for picnics by the river and to feed the ducks as the boats would glide up the river, but in my mind, on this night I would find the devil waiting for me.

I got to Marlow and parked in the car park, picked up my pouch of tobacco and the plastic white horse, and set off. I walked for about five minutes before I stood in front of a large building with huge metal shutters, and to my warped mind, they were the gates to Hell. I couldn't open the gates and became disgruntled, walking off, cursing. I was determined to face Satan and battle him if need be. I walked for miles alongside the river with no light at all except for the glow from the moon and stars. I crossed a large weir over to the other side, looking up to the stars to gauge which direction my car was. The path entered a wood; it was pitch-black and I could not see my hand in front of my face. Onwards I walked, vowing to stand up to Satan and look him in the face. I had no fear of anything – living or dead. I walked for what felt like an eternity, the small branches pressing against me until I came to a clearing with light.

At this moment, I realised the devil would not appear to me, and I cursed him. Further up the road, I stood next to a large house, called The White House, and the nameplate said the owner was a doctor. I knocked on the door, still holding my white plastic children's toy by my side. After a few minutes, a top bedroom window opened, and a man called down angrily asking what I wanted. I asked him, 'Do you have any room at the inn?' He told me to clear off or he would call the police. I was so confused as to why I had been turned away when Marion and Joseph hadn't. I was cross, tired, and very thirsty.

As I walked through a small village, I passed a couple of guys, and then I saw a hotel with its lights on. I walked in and asked very politely if I could have a glass of water. The staff member smiled and brought me a glass, then asked me what I was doing. As I sat in a plush leather chair, I told him that I was on a treasure hunt. I thanked him for the water and left, deciding it was time to head back to my car. I had walked six miles through the countryside and had no idea where I was. I ditched the toy horse on a green verge and figured out which direction I needed to go. I knew the direction because of the direction of the stars, as I had checked earlier. As I followed the road, I felt as if I were being watched from the hedges and wondered if the police or SAS were following me. It was a very long walk, but I made it back to Marlow and drove back to my dad's. I got back and, without waking Sue, cuddled up into bed with her.

When she woke in the morning, I told her what had happened and she said little. Later that day, I asked her if she would like to see where I had been, and she agreed. As we got arrived in Marlow, I began telling her bits from the night before, and as we drove through the tiny village, I told her that this was where I had left the little plastic white horse. I pulled over and picked it up. She freaked out and looked like she had seen a ghost. I now realise it was because she did not believe I had been out hiking through the Buckinghamshire countryside all night without her waking, and this was proof I had done so. I kept that silly damn horse in my wardrobe for five years until, one day, I threw it out and tried to forget the incident.

One evening, we went for a drive and ended up back at Marlow, sitting in the car park. A police car pulled up next to us and the copper, a friendly young guy, asked us for a light. He sat smoking a rollie next to us for five minutes while chatting. Afterwards, Sue turned to me and told me she was Jesus. It shocked me but, considering how I was, I do not think I was in a fit state to call her delusional. Occasionally, she asked me questions about my past and questioned whether I had been sexually abused. After a while, I believed I was. This was a false memory, which often happens in psychosis.

The next day, we went to visit our friends Carl and Winnie, who had moved close by to my dad's, running a new Dayton's Store. On the way back to my dad's, it occurred to me that my mum had made me an appointment to see the psychiatrist at Epsom Hospital, but I had no idea what date or time and I panicked. I have no idea why, but I kicked Sue out of my car and drove all the way to Surrey, to Epsom General Hospital. I walked in and soon found one of the psychiatric wards and was interviewed and given lunch. They could see I was very unwell and wanted me to stay, but I got frightened and confused and fled to my mum's. I later found out poor Sue had called Carl, who very kindly gave her a lift back to Surrey.

Sue and I chatted and decided to move to her parents'. She told me she would meet me there later that evening, and when I later walked there, an Asian lady did a similar thing as the security guard at World Dance. She had a look of death on her face and her eyes were jet-black as she walked straight for me with deathly anger, as if she were going to attack me. I believed she might have been a demon, and after seeing the shadow people, I needed little convincing.

I got to Sue's with my meagre belongings and settled in. Her house was large with old-fashioned furnishings, and her parents made me feel welcome. They knew I was ill even if I had told no one; it was so obvious by then. Sue and my mum had spoken to the local psychiatric team, who assessed me with a home visit, and they gave Sue some tablets for me to take. I later found out they were an old antipsychotic and an anti-Parkinson's drug to stop aches, pains, and involuntary movement. Not only did they not work, but I now felt the awful side effects of neuroleptic medications – I was stiff and achy with blurred vision, a foggy head, poor memory, and a plummeting IQ.

That night, I slept in the spare room, and from the outside of the window, I could hear a lot of noise, almost like the house was in a packing warehouse. I was hallucinating and hearing voices, and every time I closed my eyes, all I could see was a giant maggot. I believed it was me – that I was a giant disgusting, oozing maggot.

Sue's bedroom, it has to be said, was amazing. Picture a teenager's floor, covered in clothes, records, ornaments, and crap. She had this, but her ceiling was so artistic. Sue asked if I could sleep in her room, as she felt it would comfort me, whilst she slept in her spare room. One evening, I walked into her room and heard a voice say, 'The gas is behind the speaker . . .' I looked behind her speakers, and sure enough, there was a can of butane lighter refill gas. I became convinced that there were speakers planted around me from which I could hear voices. Even twenty-seven years later, whenever I hear a voice announcing information that I could not know, telling me where something is, I find it disturbing and unnatural.

Sue's parents decided I was not safe to be let out, so they kept the doors locked, and I felt like a prisoner. One evening at dinner, I decided that I wanted to be with Sue for the rest of my life, so I proposed. She said yes and the next day her mum took us to Croydon and she chose an engagement ring. For a moment, we felt happiness as a couple, but whilst walking back to the car, her mum said under her breath, 'Like a lamb to the slaughter.' That haunted me for years.

One afternoon, out of boredom, I sat on their stairs whilst her dad was on the phone with a family member, and I heard him tell them that there would either be a wedding or a funeral. That made me angry so much – to say it so in front of me, so coldly and bluntly.

There were many odd things that happened during my time at Sue's, like the time her parents put the TV on, and the picture was really badly distorted like the TV show was on LSD. I remember feeling it was because of me and that reality was crashing around me and everyone else, as I stopped believing in reality. It was very distressing. One evening we were sitting by her back door chatting and cuddling, and I saw a jumping spider. It jumped on me, and I believed it had climbed into my ear. I tried to get it out and, for many years after, I believed it was why I heard voices. That evening, I came across the backdoor key and made a break for freedom. I ran up to the high street and into the graveyard, not knowing where I was going. I made my way into a field with woods, and in the background, I could hear a pack of dogs like a hunt. In my mind, I was the one being hunted. I dived into the thicket of brambles and thorns. I took my ring off and threw it away, believing it to be a tracking device. My left leg had gotten caught up in the brambles and the thorns cut my calf and ankle deeply. I was a frightened man on the run from the unknown with a pack of dogs hunting me.

Nevertheless, I decided to saunter back into the field. I heard a voice saying, 'He can't go back.' Ridiculously, I walked backwards to prove the voice wrong and must have looked a proper sight to anyone who saw me. I made it back to the church, where I found Sue looking for me. She took me home and her parents looked at my leg, which was bleeding. They turned a spotlight on and I remember feeling like I was in an interrogation. The next day, about midday, Sue's dad brought me outside into the middle of the garden and put a large deckchair down for me. He handed me a large paper and told me to sit and read. It was so bizarre, but

I did as I was told for about half an hour. Then I walked around to stretch my legs; I opened the back gate and stepped out onto the pavement. The moment I stepped out, a guy dressed in shorts and a vest looked right at me, glaring, and ran towards me. I shat myself and got back into the garden to catch my breath. It was clear: I could not leave the house anymore.

The next day, my mum turned up and took me home. She told me I had an appointment at Epsom Hospital to see a consultant. They asked me to pack a small bag, and we made our way to the appointment. I walked into the psychiatric wing of the hospital and we sat in the waiting room until they called us. As I looked around, I saw what looked like a large trapdoor in the carpet with a solid metal edge. I remember thinking that if ever I was here and needed to escape, this was an option. They called us in and sat in a basic room with just a desk and chair, opposite a psychiatrist named Dr. Al Jabouri. I have no recollection of the meeting except the end, where he asked me if I would agree to be admitted and that, if not, I would be sectioned. I agreed to go in voluntarily. I would meet Dr. Al Jabouri later in life again, and he was a kind, caring man – one of the few consultants I liked.

My mum, my sister Jennine, and Sue took me up to the third floor, which consisted of two wards, Delius, and Elgar. There was an old-fashioned lounge decorated in tired peach with an old TV couch, chairs, and a fish tank. The men's ward consisted of six beds with nightstands. And then there was a room that still haunts me. It had plain white tiles, a cast-iron bath in the middle, and a large chair with restraints butted up above it. It looked like a medieval torture device, and I crapped myself. The CPN (community psychiatric nurse) touring us around turned to me and said, 'We call this the party room.'

My family left and the guy showing me around walked me back to the men's ward and said, 'I can see it in your eyes – you still have to fight.

If you need to talk, I'm here.' At the time, I was very frightened, but now I realise he meant this in a caring way.

I was shown to a bed in the empty men's ward and a female CPN asked me to go through everything I had in my small rucksack, and she wrote everything down. After she left, I sat on the bed wondering how the hell it had come to this.

Chapter Sixteen
The Ward

Being in a psychiatric ward is very frightening for so many reasons. I didn't know what to expect: Would it be violent? What medications would I be given? It was all unknown. There were about sixteen patients on my ward, Delius, and maybe the same on Elgar, each with their own problems. Some were quiet, some behaved very oddly, some were loud and scary, and a few seemed quite normal. The first few days were very confusing as I tried to fit in, and much of it was a blur. At 8:00 a.m. and 8:00 p.m., a nurse would bring a medicine trolley into the lounge, and we were all called up and given our medication. The first night he came around, I walked up and he told me I needed nothing, as I was not scared of anything, so I skulked off, thinking nothing of the odd remark.

The usual routine was a wake-up call from a nurse in the morning, then breakfast on the ground floor in a canteen. Every Monday morning, an occupational therapist would visit each of us and give us a timetable of activities for the week, which would be held in a day centre next door. I had no interest in any activities. I was not well enough and did not feel sociable. There were plenty of activities on offer, such as creative writing, woodworking, and painting, but I decided I was going to skip them all and stay in the ward's smoking room.

Lunch was in the canteen, then dinner and meds, followed by lights out at 10:00 p.m. There was a small kitchen where you could make hot drinks and there were water bottles dotted around, but the consensus was that we didn't trust that there wasn't something in the bottles to keep us quiet, so we never used them. Within a couple of days, they prescribed me a vile antipsychotic called Largactil, and its side effects were profound. It took me to a horrible place where I felt suicidal, petrified constantly, and confused; I ached all over; I lost my appetite; I became more delusional and heard voices; and I was very psychotic. If I wasn't unwell before, I was after Largactil. I turned inwards and my reality, personality, and world shrank into a small void inside of me.

On weekends, we could visit family but had to be back by Sunday night. I would spend these weekends at my nan's house, as it had much more room than my mum's house.

Sue visited me in the first few weeks and we would sit outside in the hospital garden. The garden was spotless and very peaceful, with well-kept beds and benches for people to sit. As we sat there, I looked up at the red sunset, and I remember prophesying and Sue saying that this is what I was like to someone who was sitting with us. I also remember struggling to decide if I should have a cigarette, thinking that whichever one of us smoked it would die. Nothing made sense.

I had probably been in for maybe a week when one patient called Larry approached me in the smoking room and offered to play a game with me. Larry was in his sixties, smartly dressed, yet dishevelled. He told me he had taught philosophy at Cambridge and showed me his tie. The room got crowded, as other patients became intrigued that something was happening. He told me that there had been a car boot sale in the car park that day and that he had bought some things and would like me to choose two. He produced two ruby wedding anniversary champagne flutes gilded with red glass around the stems. If I chose these, I would enjoy forty years of happy marriage with Sue, he said. He put them down and picked up the next item, an old rotary telephone. If I picked this, he said, I would always be able to contact my friends. The next item was a small lacy pink cushion with pretty lace bows tied around the top. If I chose this, I would hold the key to Sue's sexual pleasure. Last, he pulled out an old-looking scroll tied up with a ribbon. If I chose this, I would unlock the secrets of the universe and knowledge. To this day, I have no idea why I chose the way I did – maybe it was the heavy medication and the fact I was so psychotic – but I picked the telephone and the scroll. So maybe I should not be too surprised that a few days later, word got to me that Sue had left me. I look back now and wonder who would go to all the effort to invent a test for me and why. The mind boggles. For a long time, I mourned the breakup. I put Sue on a pedestal that was elevated to a ridiculous height. But she was an eighteen-year-old girl with her entire life ahead of her and her drugged-up fiancé was being held in a psychiatric ward, so I cannot blame her for leaving me. Although for many years I was very bitter, I have now accepted she had no choice.

Carl and Winnie visited me one evening, and we sat outside. He told me I would be okay; I just needed some pills. At the time, I thought he meant pilsner beer and asked him to sneak some in and hide them in the garden for me. He laughed and said OKAY. Albert and Philip also visited me once; I was sitting outside on a bench with Larry and they came and joined us. Afterwards, Larry told me that one of them was an angel and one a demon, but I never asked which was which.

Because of the Largactil, if I stood in sunlight, it burnt my skin, and 1994 was a very blistering hot summer. I do not remember being told this was a side effect, so, in my mind, I was being punished and was under the belief I was not allowed outside. I did everything possible to not go out. In my first couple of weeks, my behaviour was very odd. I kept a used condom and believed it carried the sperm of the Messiah. One day, a CPN cleared up my belongings and threw them out and I was furious at him, poor man.

The smoking room was tiny with grubby walls, eight seats, a single window, a small filthy brown extraction fan, a mirror, a table with a radio, a picture of a daffodil on the wall, a shelf of old books, and a couple puzzles. It was my home for five months. In the evenings, other patients would come in and chat and drink tea together. I had a good relationship with Larry, and we would chat about whatever it was we were psychotic about that day and believe it, even sharing delusions.

One evening, I entered the doctors' ward round room and looked at the medical books on the shelf. I picked one up, trying to find out why I was ill and looked up lead poisoning to see if my plumbing days could have made me ill. As I was reading through the book, one of the consultant doctors came in. He was an older Black man with dreadlocked hair. He told me he hoped I would enjoy my new position, and that if I ever needed drugs, that there were lots in the ward and to just ask. I took him to mean that I felt I was a doctor, as it is common for mentally ill patients to believe they hold secret jobs. As for telling me about drugs in the ward, I think they should have sacked him for negligence towards a patient, and I am so angry about this, even now.

Every Friday was a ward round. A ward round is where a large panel of about ten professionals sit in a large semicircle facing the patient and ask a myriad of questions about your mental health. There were doctors, psychologists, psychiatric nurses, occupational therapists. Every week, I sat in that chair like a rabbit caught in the headlights whilst they interrogated me. Did I hear voices, did I believe I was Jesus, etc., etc. At the time, I believed I was being interrogated, and I was damned if I was going to break. I had no reason to believe they meant me well; they were never kind or caring or showed any compassion. It was a very frightening situation for anyone, let alone someone who is psychotic and petrified of everything.

During my time in the hospital, my mum or Jennine took it in turns to visit me every night, bar weekends, for five months. Without my mum or sister, I would have had nothing and no one. Some of my former friends visited, but most did not. Instead, they vilified me. I was thrown away like cheap rubbish to be forgotten about. Every night my family came, they would bring me a packet of Benson and Hedges, as I had no money. I will never forget how hard it must have been to visit and not recognise the person I had become. And it must have been exhausting after a long day at work. My mum has told me that when she visited me, sometimes I would not talk to her and ignored her. She said I would chat to Larry in an unfamiliar language that sounded like gibberish to her. She asked me what language we were speaking, and I remember saying to her that we spoke in tongues. I asked her many years later if it seemed we were holding a conversation and not just spurting out rubbish, and she said that yes, we were.

There were lots of lovely characters I met during my time, like Kate, a girl struggling with anorexia. She was always friendly and smiling, clutching her mug of soup and struggling to swallow it. Towards the end of my stay, when I got better, I got on well with her and I wish I had stayed in contact. Another girl was in for self-harm – she was also an alcoholic. She broke out one night and took me with her. I can't remember how, but she disabled two locks, and we sneaked out for a couple of hours. She had hidden a bottle of vodka up a tree and retrieved it, and we went for a walk around the grounds whilst she got drunk.

The World Cup was on during my stay and a lot of us would sit around the TV if our teams were playing. The funny thing was that we all thought we could control the match by moving certain parts of our body. So, if one of our players got the ball, I would twitch my foot to make sure he scored. I imagine the staff laughed at us all sitting there twitching in front of the football matches, thinking we had special powers.

After a few months, Larry, Kate, and I were given private rooms, which was nice. But it was still very lonely, and staff would wander by every so often and lift the outside shutter on the door window to check on us, which meant we had no privacy. I remember lying in bed one night very lonely and needing a hug, and reaching out to Kate next door with my arm. I may be wrong, but I remember getting up and walking out of my room, only to be ushered back into mine. I only ever wanted a hug.

Every patient in the ward had a delegated nurse who looked after you and monitored you. Mine was an extremely attractive girl my age, Eli, who did not speak to me once in five months. I never saw that girl smile. Why she was a nurse is beyond me; she had the compassion of a wet fish.

One day, my mum visited and told me to have a bath, as I was very neglectful of my hygiene. I asked for my razor, which the nurses kept so we could not harm ourselves. I went into the bathroom and lay in the hot bath while a CPN called Claire sat outside the door. I shaved, and during every stroke of my razor, she would say, 'Ow.' I have no idea how, but I felt I was being gaslighted; she wasn't very pleasant.

At some point during the five months, I became very suicidal. I walked to the top flight of the stairs and wanted to hurl myself down, but it petrified me that the demons were waiting for me on the other side, and I felt trapped and terrified. So, I starved myself. I did not eat for two weeks, even when my family brought me a delicious McDonald's; I just wanted it all to end. None of them realised that I was not drinking except for twice a day when I took my meds and was given the tiny container of water to wash down the pills. After two weeks, a lovely lady who had lost her son and was in for depression pulled me to one side. She told me he had fallen into the River Thames and drowned, and she did not want me to die either. It was a very heartfelt plea, and I found myself torn, but she was so genuine that I listened to her and took her advice and began eating again.

After five months, the head CPN, a lovely man named Barry, came to me and told me he wanted to try me on a different medication called Depixol. He told me it was an intramuscular injection and was administered every two weeks. Within two days, the darkness lessened, and I talked more. For the first time in a very long time, I felt like a human being, not a tortured soul. I have to ask myself why it took five months of being on an awful antipsychotic medication that was not working for them to change my meds. I would assume that, after trying a medication for a couple of months, if there is no improvement, you try something else. I don't believe this was an oversight; I think it was disgraceful neglect by the doctors. I could have been well with in half that time had they done their job. Even to this day, I feel like I was a guinea pig in some kind of shitty experiment. The thing I found the hardest during my stay was that nobody in the ward cared. No one came up to me and sat next to me and tried to talk to me. I think all I wanted was a hug. I had hope, though – and that kept me going – that one day I would fall in love again and be hugged.

Chapter Seventeen
Release

A week after my Depixol injection, I was finally discharged and moved back home to my mums in Banstead. It was an immense relief for me and my mum, although my confidence was smashed. None of my friends wanted to know me at all, and I had no one to go out and socialise with. The friends I once knew ignored me. My little sister, Melanie, had a few friends who befriended me and were so kind. They were younger, did not do drugs, and were quite clean-cut. We would meet in another local pub called The Wheatsheaf in Banstead, and would play pool, drink, and chat. I was always very grateful to them for their kindness when others turned their backs on me.

My mum was working for Petra Fina at the time in their Epsom office and was asked if she would put an exchange student up for a few months and bring her into work. My mum obliged and soon welcomed a sweet Dutch girl, Marie Suzanne. I was thrown out of my large bedroom the night before and given back the box room. During the night, I got up, naked, and went to use the toilet. Out of habit, instead of walking to my new box room, I walked into my old large room – yes, the room that Marie Suzanne was now sleeping in. Half asleep, I walked over to the bed and looked down to see Marie looking up at me stark naked. I came to and rushed back to my room. The next night, I took her to the local pub, and I explained that her room was in fact my old room. I was very embarrassed when I asked if she saw my bits. She replied yes; she had. Marie stayed with us for four or five months and socialised with both me and my mum. It was obvious she liked me, but I was a bit damaged and she wasn't my type, either, although she was a spit for Sophia Loren.

I wasn't well enough to go back to university but needed routine and some money, so I began looking around for a job. I spoke to Mike, who told me he had left Dayton's and was now working for Bridge's in Cheam. Bridge's was a tiny food store but had everything a person needed. Cheam, a small village in Surrey, was only a fifteen-minute drive away, so I went for a chat with him and met some of his colleagues. Mike told me he was looking for someone to run the grocery section, which meant all the ordering of dry goods and putting out deliveries every day. They offered me the job, and I was soon working hard every day, throwing myself into work again. It was very humdrum, but when you put your back into it and took pride in it, it was fun. The first couple of months were fine, but then that bastard of a demon cannabis came back to haunt me. I had been med-free for some time, so I thought I would be okay smoking a bit of hash. My psychosis swiftly returned, and I hid it from everyone again. I knew I was suffering but would not tell anyone. It was my secret. Mike soon received a promotion to a much bigger store, and we found ourselves with a new manager who I do not believe smiled once during my time working for him. He took me off the grocery department and put me on the tiny delicatessen. He'd decided he was going to look after the grocery ordering. I was very displeased to be serving a dozen people a day on a ten-foot deli. But I made the most of it and gave away free samples. The department ran a huge profit because of a trick I had learnt called 'buying in'. When a large ham goes on promotion at half price, I would buy four more and store them, and once the promotion finished, I sold it hard at full price and made a lot. As long as dates were regularly checked and nothing out of date was sold, it was fine. One day, the profit and loss sheet came in and the manager asked me how the hell I was doing it. I explained, and I got a bollocking and was told not to do it again. It was quite amusing, because they were his P and L figures, and he wanted to make them look shit.

There was a lovely girl who ran the cash office, Hailey. She was my age, taught ballet to children, and was quite attractive. We got on well, and I flirted with her once and she gave the tomboy 'Ew, boys' reply, so I didn't bother again. During my time at Bridge's, I caught quite a few shoplifters. It was always joints of meat or alcohol. I noticed their body language and just watched them. When they had passed the checkouts without paying, I jumped on them. I always let them go and just banned them from the store. Hailey approached me one day and told me we had a thief on the tills, taking out a tenner here and there. The problem was, on a usual day, maybe five or six staff members could use a checkout, so proving who it was, was very difficult, but we had a plan. Every day we wrote who was in and which till was used and when money went missing. It was quite a straightforward process of elimination. So, on a day when £10 went messing, everyone not working that day was taken off the wanted list. We only had one name in the end, and we questioned her, and she admitted her crimes and was sacked. I felt Hailey and I did a superb job catching her.

I had some tough days in Bridge's with my mental health. Music played over the Tannoy, and I believed it was referring to me. One afternoon I went up to the staff room for a coffee and a cigarette, but I could not figure out which hand to smoke with – my left or right. In my mind, I had a biblical delusion going on with using hands for different things. The assistant manager picked up a cigarette and placed it in her right hand and lit it. And I followed suit. I was incredibly grateful to her for that. Mike settled into his new store in Shepperton and asked if I wanted to go over with him and work in the produce department. I had heard it was a terrible department in Shepperton and that it was losing money and not performing well, so I jumped at the chance. They placed me in the Chessington Bridge's to learn the ropes for two weeks and I enjoyed my time there. All the staff were nice; it was quite close; the manager was kind; and I had a crush on one assistant. The manager said to me occasionally he would like me to stay, but I had stars in my eyes for Shepperton, so I declined each time.

I found myself at Shepperton Bridge's at 6:15 every morning and not finishing until 6:30 at night. It was a long drive, too, at fifty minutes each way, and I put my heart and soul into that job. The produce section was large, and I only had part-time help from an older lady and it was short-staffed. Not only did I have to get the stock in and put it out on display, but I had to check all the fruit and vegetables to see if they were out of date and then reduce or write them off. There was daily ordering according to how much had been sold that day as well. It was chaos, and twelve hours a day would not cut it. I became unwell again and was paranoid, anxious, stressed, and delusional. My thoughts were confused, and I felt like a child in an adult's world. I told Mike I was struggling, and he told me to order stock a certain way, and then the deputy manager would come down and tell me to order a different way. I was not well enough to hold a meeting with them both, as they were both pulling at me in different directions. I was burned out and soon left.

During a drunken night out with my wonderful mate Neil, we ended up chatting to a couple of girls in a bar. After the bar closed, we drove to Box Hill, my old motorbike haunt. I ended up with one of them, a girl named Sophie who both Neil and I agreed was a babe. We had a little rough tumble on the grass, and the other girl grabbed hold of Neil. As we dropped them off later that night, I tried to get Sophie's number, as we had seemed to click, but she would not give it out, saying she had a boyfriend. I eventually teased where she worked out of her, and after some digging a couple of days later, I called her. We began an odd fling that lasted about three months. She lived an hour away by the coast and I would go down and stay the night whilst her boyfriend worked nights. She would also visit her friend in Surrey and we would meet up with them. I liked Sophie, but our relationship was never loving; it was a fling. I am unsure if I ever believed she had a boyfriend, as I never saw proof of a guy living there. He never called her, and she was never nervous about being caught. After three months, she called it off and told me she was making a go at being with him. For all I know, she had met someone else.

My mum had moved to a lovely new three-bedroom house in Walton-on-the-Hill called Pond Farm Close. It was so very idyllic. My nan lived in the first house, and we lived in the fifth. All the residents of the close got on well and it was a real mix of characters. I spent a lot of time with my nan, with whom I was close. If I was broke, I would ask her if she had any jobs to do, and she would have me doing some gardening and give me £10 or £20. She was so very good to me, and I loved my nan.

My mum met a guy who worked on the site, Philip. He was the painter and decorator, and soon he had moved in. Philip was the stereotype of a builder, common and crass. I disliked him immediately, although everyone else loved his cheeky charm. One day, I was off work and dozing on the sofa. My new brother-in-law, Adel, was there, and Philip walked in and yelled at me to get off the sofa. I stood up and told him to fuck off, that this was not his place and it was my day off. He yelled back, and I went for him, but my brother-in-law pulled me back. I knew Philip was a no-good piece of shit from that moment onwards, but it seemed as if I was the only one who saw it.

The neighbour to our left, Steve, was a stockbroker. He was young, rich, arrogant, drove a flashy bright red TVR, and took drugs in his hot tub with young women. I was jealous of him and his position. He was good-looking and could charm the socks off everyone. Every night before bed, I would smoke some cannabis. It made me feel as if it wrapped me up in cotton wool and gave me a warm feeling, and it helped me sleep. One evening, I was lying in bed and heard two female voices. It sounded like they were coming from outside, maybe thirty feet away. They were talking about Odour Eaters, which are innersoles for your shoes. It was bizarre, and the next day I bought some out of curiosity. I did not think of them as voices. It was not long before these voices became a problem. Steve the stockbroker blasted music out; I began hearing the two female voices who I believed were from next door, too. I was desperate to get away from next door but did not tell anyone what was going on. I called my dad and asked if I could come to stay with him a while and look for work there. He agreed, and so I moved to High Wycombe, saying goodbye to my mum and her arsehole boyfriend, Philip.

I soon found a job in a small office reselling software used by construction companies. The money was nothing special, and on the surface, the company looked 'shiny' but it was not. We had to cold call clients using the Yellow Pages and try to get appointments for our salesperson to go out and sell the software. There were two of us, and we never even got to see it in action. Even though I asked for an overview to explain the software's merits to potential clients, we were told no, keep calling. The atmosphere in the office was quite dire, and the work was soulless. Most of the men wore suits, but I did not have a suit, so my dad lent me one of his. I did not have any other option; it was a very old-fashioned Farah suit. The other salesperson there was seeing the receptionist and took the piss out of Farah's, but I kept quiet, knowing I could not afford a suit. I was crushed with embarrassment. I remember driving to work one morning and my voices were relentless, and I was half crying and half screaming at them to leave me alone. They taunted me: 'Diddum's, poor Darren.' I felt an inner turmoil that nobody knew about, and I told no one. Inside, I was screaming to be released from my captors torturing me. After four or five months, I had been through my telephone books and asked what to do next and was told to leave. They just hired another robot who started at page one again. In my time there, nobody had got an appointment. What amateurs.

During the few months I worked at the software company, I didn't know anyone, so I drove up to the old village I grew up in as a kid, Studley Green, and paid a visit to the pub, The Kings Arms, where I bought a drink. The pub was quite busy and there were a few people my age playing pool, so I began chatting to them. One girl stood out, as she was very assertive and attractive. I met with them a few times and got it on with her one night, but it was like sleeping with a corpse, as she just lay there. I don't know if she had a history of abuse, but I would not have been surprised. We saw each other for a little while longer, but there was nothing there, and they were all stoners. I had some pot one night whilst the film The Mask was on, and it freaked me out and gave me an unpleasant episode for the night. After that, we drifted and I tried calling her, but I got the 'she is out' treatment.

I was struggling so badly with my psychosis and I finally realised I needed help, so I called my old mental health team and was put through to the lovely Dr. Al Jabouri, the original consultant who had admitted me. He made an appointment with me a week later.

At the appointment, for the very first time, I admitted to him and the lady CPN there that I was hearing voices. He told me not to worry and that; the CPN, Hema, would give me a Depixol injection and I would feel better within a day or so. I still remember her asking me if I wanted to get better, and that if I did, it would take a lot of effort. She encouraged me to give up cannabis and said that if I needed anything to have a glass of red wine in the evening. She was my first community-based psychiatric nurse and was lovely and caring.

I moved everything back to my mum's. I told her I was hearing voices and she yelled at me that it was not true and was cross with me.

My dad had booked a holiday for us both. It was not my cup of tea, but I had not been away for years, so I accepted. It was two weeks on the Peloponnese on the Greek mainland to go windsurfing. I did a few lessons at a sailing lake, but I did not take to it. Being out of work and having my holiday three weeks away, I needed money, so I signed up at an agency. They called at six every morning and told me where to go and what I was doing. I spent three weeks sweeping the streets in Mitcham in London. It was simple work, if dull, but I felt very proud that many people would not demean themselves by sweeping roads and would rather collect the dole, but I had chosen this work instead. Three weeks later, my dad and I were on the Peloponnese. I hated windsurfing, as I was terrible at it and spent my entire time in the water. My dad had spent a lot of time on the boards and sailed, so he found it very easy. Halfway through the holiday, I put my back out and was in an awful lot of pain. I struggled to move around, so I spent a week laid up in bed. I found a little friend in a very loving ginger cat who cuddled up to me every day until we left. When I got home, I immediately searched for meaningful work.

Chapter Eighteen
Work

In 1995, I saw an advert for a deputy manager in Shoe Zoo in nearby Epsom, so I applied. A week later, I was called into an interview in Epsom with the area manager, a pleasant guy named Martin. I was really nervous so I asked for a glass of water, then had an anxiety attack. I told Martin, and he gave me ten minutes to gather myself and come back, and it all went well. They offered me the job. I thought it was decent of him to give me a chance considering how I was in the interview. A couple of days later, I turned up, was given my Shoe Zoo T-shirt, and introduced myself to everyone. The manager was a nice girl about my age, Deborah; she was firm but fair. She knew her job well and was happy to teach me as I went along. There were quite a few younger members of staff, and all were good fun. One of my first jobs was to stock the children's shoes, and they partnered me with a bubbly girl named Cath. As we worked, we chatted away, and she was so easy to talk to. A lady walked in and began looking at the shoes maybe eight feet away from us, and she bent down to look on the bottom shelf and let rip a massive fart. Well, I went into a fit of hysterics and had to walk into the back room, unable to contain myself. Cath soon followed and was laughing her head off with me, and at how I was belly laughing so hard. We had tears in our eyes, and from that moment onwards, Cath and I got on like a house on fire.

Being the assistant manager, I had to delegate work to the staff but always helped them. If there is one thing I dislike, it is a manager who delegates and walks away. Even working with the staff for a short time shows good leadership. Managers who lead by example earn more respect and loyalty from everyone.

It was soon Christmas, and the store opened on a Sunday to welcome in more trade. They called only two of us in the first week, and the high street was dead. There was not much to do, as they had all done it the previous day. The girl I worked with was named Hazel. Even though she was much younger than me, I found her very attractive. She did not stop talking. As we stood in the empty shop, very bored, I gave her £10 and sent her over to Argos over the road to buy a board game. She went off and twenty minutes later returned with a game called Kerplunk. We sat on the shop floor for three hours playing Kerplunk and talking bollocks. From that moment onwards, Hazel would tell people how she'd met her boss and we would end up being wonderful friends.

I learnt the ropes quickly in the Epsom branch down to Deborah's teaching and began helping at different stores that were going through makeovers. One of our flagship stores was closed in Croydon High Street and having a huge refit. I spent a lot of time helping replan the shelves and organising vast amounts of stock. The stores had a great team spirit and worked well, with everyone mucking in and working late. It was whilst working in the Croydon store one day with Deborah and a team of maybe twelve others that I was told Deborah had a crush on me and they teased us. I felt embarrassed. She was a nice, quiet girl but did nothing for me, and I felt guilty. And I did not even feel ready for any kind of relationship. When we returned to our Epsom Store, I felt a little embarrassed and awkward.

We had a lot of fun in store with the staff. During our own refit, we had to take all the shoes in the store out of the boxes and store them upstairs in our large stockroom. All you could see were thousands of boxes piled up halfway to the ceiling. One day, whilst in a silly mood, I called the younger staff up to watch, and I dived headfirst into the vast pile, much to their amusement. Before long, they were all throwing themselves into cardboard shoe boxes. It was nice for them to have a little fun, as we all worked hard for Deborah.

Things at home were difficult with my mum and Philip. He made my life quite challenging, and my mum was smitten, so she didn't see it. He poisoned her against me at every opportunity. One day, she told me there was a small flat being rented in Redhill above her hairdresser's. It was tiny and basic but would do me good. In all fairness to Philip, he went in and slapped some paint on the walls before I moved in. The rent was £400 a month, and I signed up for six months. I paid for electricity with a meter which took fifty pence pieces. I was taking home £650 a month, so I had £250 for everything. The night I moved in, my good friend Neil and I went out for an Indian and a pint, and I did not go out again for six months. The flat was freezing cold, dark, and very dreary. I had an oil chip fryer, and every night for dinner, I ate fried oven chips and a tin of chicken curry. Money was so tight, I did not have electricity, and my lovely nan would save up her fifty pence coins for me. I remember lying in bed very depressed, cold and lonely, and feeling desperate as I took my Stela zine antipsychotic. 'Will life ever improve?' I asked myself. After my six months' lease was up, I asked my mum if I could move back home and she agreed, although it was not long before an argument started about me living there. She told me I should save and buy a flat. I was so furious that I vowed I would save my arse off, and within a couple of years I had saved £2,500, which was enough for a deposit towards my flat. It was my anger that focused me to save so hard.

Within eight months of working at the Epsom store, I was asked if I would like to take on my store in Caterham, a small town outside of

South London. It was a tiny quiet store, but a foot up the ladder, and I accepted. The first couple of days there, I went through the staff rota and checked all the systems were in place for it to run smoothly. Whilst going through the office and safe, I found a bag of cash that had not been banked. It contained £750 and had been sitting there for over a week unbanked. I called the head office, who made a note and told me to bank it. I was sure then and even now that this was a test of my honesty. It was not the first time I had found a sizable amount of cash at work, and being honest anyway, it was never a problem.

There were maybe five members of staff, and I wanted to know how each one worked – their attitude, loyalty, strengths, and weaknesses. There was one full-time young guy who was pleasant, did what he was told, but was not career minded. To him, this was just a job. We had a young student who was very immature and obnoxious. He would open and close the till to print out twenty blank receipts just to make paper chains. I explained to him why this was an issue, not only for security reasons, and he did not take it on board, so at the earliest opportunity, I got rid of him. Another student in college had an attitude at being told what to do and often called in sick. After a couple of sickies, I began making a note of her sick dates and her excuses, and after six weeks, I sacked her. Her mother called up spitting feathers, so I explained her behaviour and she did not believe her daughter was like that, so I went through my diary and put the phone down, pleased I had recorded it. I began recruiting and took on two young girls eager for work. Another girl, Veronica, had worked at the store before she had gone to university and so she knew the work. She asked if she could work during her summer break and we welcomed her on board.

The work was slow, so I needed self-motivation to keep the stock clean and organised. We had two large deliveries a week which needed going through, checking, and the packing paper taken out of each box before being put out for the customers in size order and to plan. Serving customers on the checkout, helping customers with their choice and size and banking, and then a good tidy up was about it. Standing in a small shoe shop in a small village with a small footfall, it would have been easy to have been bored out of one's mind, but as mentioned before, being motivated to keep busy was a must.

I socialised a lot with the Epsom staff I had worked with and became friends with two girls who worked with me at Caterham. Hazel from Epsom and I became good friends, and we chilled occasionally, just listening to music. I didn't feel as though I was compromising my position at work in Caterham, as we all had a healthy respect for one another and they were loyal staff and friends. One night I was out with Laura and Veronica. We had gone out to a pub for a few drinks, and Laura told me that Veronica fancied me and she wanted me to kiss her. I was nervous, almost anxious. We got it together and spent a lovely three months dating whilst she was back from university. Veronica was a small, slim girl with a short blonde bob. She had a strong jaw, and everyone told me how pretty she was. She had the most beautiful lips and a smile that melted my heart. About a week before she returned to uni, I broached the subject of my condition and the fact I was on meds to keep me stable. She immediately asked if it was to do with dopamine, and I told her yes it was. And that was the last I saw of her. I tried to call her before she went but was told she was out. I wanted to continue our relationship whilst she was at uni, but it was not to be. It quite upset me that, even though she knew me, as soon as I mentioned medication for mental health, she'd run a mile. This just made me very wary of whom I told and reinforced the stigma that went with mental illness. It hurt as much as being unwell.

About a month before Veronica left – and I was still dating her – Laura and I were working alone in the store. We had cover come in, and we both headed downstairs to our little kitchen for lunch. As we walked down the stairs, Laura turned to me and asked me if she could give me a blow job, like asking if I wanted a cup of coffee. I was quite taken aback and confused. I thanked her and declined. I was dating one of her friends, and she herself was a dear friend at the time. Also, what is it with girls randomly asking if they could suck my dick? I cannot fathom what is so magical about my dick. Imagine if the tables were turned and I asked a female colleague if I could go down on her – they would have branded me a pervert, a sex pest, and I would have been sacked on the spot.

We got word one day that our holding company, the British Shoe Corporation, was folding and closing 95 percent of its stores. They offered us £500 if we stayed on to the grisly end, but I started looking and got a head start. The full-time guy I had there landed a job at a large computer shop in Croydon as a salesperson, and his money was much better than I was getting, so I applied, too. After a couple of interviews, they offered me the same job. The week before I handed my store over to the area manager, we blitzed it, and I can say it was immaculate. When I handed the keys over, he looked at me open-mouthed and I told him I wanted to go out with a good reputation, giving 110 percent until I left.

☒

Chapter Nineteen
Computer Land

In 1996, at twenty-seven, I began working at the flagship store of Computer Land in Croydon. It was the first computer store set up by a husband-and-wife team, and they did so well that a large well-known group bought them out and rolled out many new stores around the UK. I worked with them for a year and a half, and everything about it was enjoyable. After my induction, they gave me a training manual/programme to follow. During the day, I was free to go study as long as we weren't short-staffed. The training was very thorough, involved multiple media sources, and was very well thought-out, including an extensive course in sales. After I completed it, I would mentor others, giving presentations and guidance on techniques used. The money was so much better than Shoe Express and doubled to £1,200 a month.

For the first six months, I was just a regular salesperson selling desktop computers according to the customer's needs. We were heavily targeted on selling the warranty that was in use, but because everything we sold, including the warranty, paid commission, we pushed hard. I do not think I could have sold it had I not believed in its merits; having a belief in something you sell is necessary. During my first Christmas in the store, we were incentivised to sell certain items and sell value. They paid us bonuses in vouchers that could be spent in most of the high street. A few of us cottoned on to the fact that a very good printer paid an incentive of £25 per sale. And so, I printed up a high-quality photograph from it on excellent paper and stood with it in a folder by the printers for two weeks. After Christmas, I had earned over £600 in vouchers and bought a lovely suit and outfit from Next. Soon after that, I was told I was being promoted to a senior sales position. This meant I received a small pay increase, supervised the other staff, and stood in for the shop floor manager (SFM) if the staff needed managing. There were some interesting people at work from all different backgrounds – a lot of students, and some mature people who just wanted a break or were stuck for work. There were your obvious cliques, but I got on with most, barring a couple of obnoxious, self-entitled rich kids who hated discipline. I became good friends with one manager who, it turned out, was shagging two of the young female staff, and both of the women were taken.

There was a lovely little cafe in the store's front for customers and staff during breaks to go grab a coffee or a bacon sandwich. I was told that one girl serving was getting married in a few months and wanted one last fling in the form of me. She was an attractive girl and quite busty, nice to chat to, but I turned it down. I did not want to be the person who might ruin a couple's marriage, and I thought it a terrible thing to do to a fiancé. The staff at the cafe reminded me daily of this and it became embarrassing, but I got huge portions of food out of it.

As time went on, they offered me another promotion to shop floor manager (SFM). This was a deputy manager position, and it thrilled me. It was a position that commanded respect, was still quite hands-on with the staff, and I had some free rein to implement changes. I handled forty-five sales staff; most were part-time. My role involved standing at the head of the sales department and organising my staff. During the week after Christmas, we opened on Boxing Day and the start of the sales. The store was packed with members of the public, and I felt like a musical conductor arranging an orchestra of salespeople helping the hundreds of the public trying to buy the latest computer but not knowing about them. I helped with customer complaints, including some screamers, and arranging stock displays. One afternoon, we had to arrange over one hundred packages of software, and I arranged them in a giant circle rising into a spiral the higher it went up. I was told half an hour after we finished it and we were all admiring our artistic talents that it did not leave enough room for wheelchairs and was a hazard and to take it down.

I went through all the sales figures for the last quarter and looked for room for improvement. There was an enormous hole in the sale of consumable items, like cables and ink cartridges. I set about training the staff on upselling and set targets, sitting them down regularly for one-to-ones to discuss their progress. I was so happy when the figures came in and the sales were so much higher, and the staff took the incentive on board and embraced the push.

I began property hunting, and because of my pay increase, I had saved £2,500 towards a deposit. I found a studio flat at the top end of Sutton in a lovely location in a small block. It was a new build and whilst basic, it was homely. I arranged the mortgage and moved in. I was still socialising with some of my old Shoe Zoo friends, in particular Hazel's boyfriend, a younger guy, Mitch. He was not the sort of person I would usually be friends with, as he was an arrogant jack, the lad, but he could charm anyone. Maybe I was lonely, but for whatever reason we hit it off and became friends. We were hanging out with a friend of a friend named Donna, who was a single mother living in a small council flat, and one of her friends, Cath. Both were lovely girls, and we had some fun times.

Our Christmas do was held in The Chicago Rock Cafe in Sutton, which we had hired out for one very long drunken night of shots and eighties Christmas dance music. Everyone was given a certain number of plastic tokens to hand in at the bar for drinks, and for some odd reason, they gave me the job of looking after them. I made a lot of friends that night, as I handed out handfuls of tokens whilst telling people, 'This is strictly between me and you.'

One night I went out with Matt, the deputy manager who was shagging anything he could whilst married with a baby. We ended up very drunk at some girls' flat nearby. The two of them both fancied him and were both trying it on with him. I ended up as his loyal wingman, trying to fix him up with the attractive one, whilst trying to get anything I could from the other one. Matt and the attractive one disappeared for ten minutes, and the ugly one who had tried to lay claim to him went looking for them. I followed her out and into the bedroom, and she walked in on him having his dick sucked. She went apeshit and began ranting at her friend and then kicked us out. He would often laugh, as she was a police woman, and would joke about how he got a blowie off a copper.

Things had gotten dry for me, and I felt the need for some affection and a good seeing-to. I went out determined to pull, even if she was uglier than a bulldog chewing a wasp. I met a girl named Amy, got a snog, and swapped numbers. We met the next night for a drink in Wimbledon where she worked, and I saw her for a short while. We dated for about six weeks. She led a sheltered life, and I did not mean to hurt her. After we split up, she began dating a guy from her work, and I was pleased for her.

During the last six months of my time at Computer Land, there was an enormous problem with insider theft. Small items worth a lot of money were being taken out of 'the cage', such as software disks and small electrical items. In all honesty, I did not pay any attention to it, as we always had two security guards on every day with their own room and CCTV, and if they could not figure it out, even after searching us going in and out of the store, how was I going to solve it?

I answered to three deputy managers and the general manager, who was aloof and chatted little. My main line manager was an unusual guy named Arron. He invited me over to his for dinner one night cooked by his Italian wife, who did not speak a word of English. He asked me what I liked and did not, and I told him I hated fish and pasta. I arrived with a bottle of wine and sat down and was given herb-baked pasta balls in a fish broth. I was horrified and pushed it around the bowl for half an hour, occasionally trying miniscule portions without throwing up. Arron began giving me weekly appraisals and started busting my balls about petty things, and I got fed up week in week out, but I wasn't the sort to go to the unsociable general manager who never spoke. So, I became unhappy at work. As luck would have it, the company next door to us, a large sofa warehouse, headhunted me. I have no idea how they got my number, but the area manager was quite insistent on chatting to me, and with the crap going on with Arron, I eventually went along. As I sat on one of the sofas, chatting with the area manager, he explained how amazing they were, how they were expanding and needed future managers, and I was just what they were after. He offered me a £10K pay raise as deputy manager in Croydon and told me I would be trained up during my time there, first in Thurrock in Kent to learn the basics, and then in-store. I was twenty-nine at the time, and a £10K pay raise was a vast amount. I just saw pound signs in my eyes. I went to my general manager and handed in my notice. He told me that furniture sales were very dull, with the week being dead and then crazy busy at weekends, but I had made my mind up.

I bumped into an old member of staff from Computer Land many years later whilst out shopping, and he told me he had thought that the store thief was Arron. He had seen him in the stockroom cage handling an expensive digital camera, and then the next day it was stolen. He went to the general manager and told him what he had seen, but he was brushed off and nothing was ever done. He had then heard that six months later, Arron had bought three laptops with a cheque that was not guaranteed, and they never saw him again. He didn't give any notice and fled the country, moving back to Italy with his wife. And that was how they found out who the long-term thief was. He held all the keys and was trusted and respected too much, and that was the company's downfall. I have wondered in hindsight if he was giving me a hard time or if he was trying to manage me out because of his thieving.

Chapter Twenty
Sofas

Before joining my cheap sofa store in Croydon, South London, I spent a month in Thurrock learning the basics on how to sell sofas and the ridiculous cash-claim-back scheme that gave you cash back. It was so complicated and exploited a loophole in the company's finance terms, and if followed to the letter, the customer got cash back. We pushed that loophole so hard that when customers asked about interest-free credit, we told them we did one better and gave them free money. The other service we pushed hard was a spray that went on the sofa to make it easier to clean spills.

When I got into the swing of things, I was close to the top of being one of the best sellers with a sell rate of 97 percent, and it annoyed every single salesperson in my store, who swore I used to lie, which I did not; I just believed in it 100 percent. I soon learnt that if you snooze, you lose in sales, and it was very, very competitive. If I walked away from someone for five minutes during a sale, they were fair game, and it pissed me off. The management would encourage this, for obvious reasons. They wanted us not just hungry for sales, but ravenous. This built up some drama in some stores between people, but we were told to do the same to them.

I returned to the Croydon store under the manager, Philip, who was a complete muppet and did not teach me anything about what he did. Every morning, we would hold a brief for thirty minutes before the store opened. This would comprise various training techniques and how to overcome objections that customers would say to us when trying to sell something. We had an answer to counter most situations that were not in our favour. Within a couple of months, I began taking these sessions most days and quite enjoyed them. I recruited two members of staff who were customers, and because of that, they were quite loyal to me. We had three women who were lovely, and I found out years later that two of them had had the hots for me and would argue with each other over me. I never realised and was shocked, but I laughed when one of them told me. Apparently, I had Brad Pitt hair going on. There were a few guys in the stockroom whom we did not mix with, one salesperson who was an angry bully, and one on the cash desk. The store was like a morgue during the week, and then Saturday morning until closing time Sunday, we did not stop. There was no job satisfaction, as there was no team cohesion from the manager, and everyone was angry.

One day, Hailey, a girl from another store, came to pick up a mattress from us for a customer at her store. She flirted with me and used her feminine charm and within a week, she called me and we went out for a drink. I was told by some staff in my store not to go, as they knew her as 'psycho' in her store. I laughed it off, and it is one of my biggest regrets.

Chapter Twenty-One
Hailey

Hailey was a short and slim brunette with shoulder-length curly hair and wore thick glasses. We began dating in 1999, making me twenty-nine and Hailey a few years younger. It was not long before she began staying over at my flat occasionally, although she had a very large flat herself in Lewisham, where we sometimes stayed. We had a rocky start when, one day whilst I was at work, she went through my drawers and found my journal. I had been advised to write one by my CPN to gauge how I felt and how my symptoms were. She read every single bit, and when I got home, she confronted me. I was furious at her going through my personal effects. I was aghast that she could search my room, looking for anything that personal. We had only been dating a short time, and it was my choice when and what I said about my diagnosis. It was an invasion of my privacy. We rowed, and she moved her stuff out. Hailey left her job and began working as a local estate agent. She dated a guy in her office, but a couple of weeks later, we reconciled. I was never happy that she continued to work with him and always had my doubts.

One day whilst I was at work, I had a call from Hailey telling me she had been involved in a car crash. I went to visit her in the hospital, but she only had cuts and bruises. When we got home, she told me something that shocked me to the core. She had been tested at the hospital and was told she was pregnant. I was fuming. She'd told me she was on the pill, and whilst there is a small percentage of women on the pill who get pregnant, I suspected foul play, and later in our relationship I realised she had likely planned it and not taken contraception, hoping to trap me. I had never wanted children because I always felt I was too selfish. I enjoy my own time, and giving my time up to a baby at three a.m. was not my idea of fun. I was also very cautious about passing my condition on to any child. Later in life, I am obviously very glad I have my children but just wish I had had a choice.

The week before the turn of millennium, Hailey caught the flu and was poorly. I spent what should have been a memorable evening celebrating the turn of a new millennium, the year 2000, looking after her. I did not begrudge this then but do now. Afterwards, we had a silly argument, and she insisted I apologise to her, even though I felt I was right. She moved back to her flat in Ladywell, and a week later, she called me. She told me I should apologise to her and buy her flowers and some chocolates or she would go to my manager at my work and tell him I had a diagnosis of schizophrenia. I was so bloody angry at her blackmail but also fearful of losing my job. I gave my manager, Philip, the benefit of the doubt and hoped my standing in the store outweighed the horrible stigma that surrounds mental illness. He seemed indifferent. A week later, I was informed my performance was not up to standard and that I was to be given a formal last warning. He had two representatives with him during the 'trial' and I argued my case well, telling him I knew it was because of what I had revealed to him. He told me it had nothing to do with the decision and came from the area manager. It was, of course, a setup to manage me out, and I was so upset and angry. I knew I maybe had two weeks before any tiny indiscretion had me kicked out, and so I looked for a new job.

The area manager of another popular local sofa company came in and took a seat, pretending to be a customer. I approached him, not knowing he was with the other company, and he asked me why he should buy from us when the other sofa company was offering interest-free credit with nothing to pay for a year. I explained to him the silly loophole we used against the finance company and said, 'What could be better than interest-free credit than being given free money?' I received a few phone calls from him at work after he left, and he told me who he was and took my home number so we could chat. A couple of interviews in the Croydon store went very well. I had the gift of the gab and our previous chat had given me a lot of credit with him, so they offered me a position.

I spent a few weeks training in various stores and learning the ropes before being placed in the Maidstone store. The staff were nice and my manager, Isaac, treated me very well. The guys were fun to work with, and of course, the weekend was frantic. My sales figures were not the highest in store, but respectable.

Hailey and I talked a lot, and rather than walk away, I did what I felt was the decent thing with her being pregnant, making a go of things even though she was a nightmare to be around and we had with frequent arguments. We decided to both sell our flats and buy a new house we could call ours. I had made £24K in profit, and Hailey, £76K. The home we bought was a five-bedroom terrace in Bexleyheath, an area I did not know, in Kent just outside of London. It made travelling to work for me easier, though, and I guess it was a fresh start. I cannot remember how much we paid, but it never felt like home to me. Hailey had proposed to me, but the first time I refused. Our son, Daniel, was born on 29 July 2000. Hailey had a caesarean, and I was in the theatre with her, although hiding behind the top end of the curtain, as seeing blood and guts was not my thing. The nurse cleaned Daniel up and passed him to me. As I cradled him in my arms, he opened his eyes and just looked at me. I held him for five minutes, and it was the most moving experience in my life, barring one other. A few days later, he was back home with us. That year he slept maybe two hours a night, and even though I worked, I sat up with him rocking him, exhausted, and then worked like a zombie each day. Hailey told me she had him during the day, so it was down to me to have him at night whilst she slept. I think this is one reason Daniel and I are so close now.

Hailey proposed again, and reluctantly and foolishly, I agreed. Hailey had decided she wanted the wedding to be on Valentine's Day, which has ruined every Valentine's Day for me since, but that's another story. We spent months planning our day with a vintage Rolls-Royce and a matching Daimler for the bridesmaids. She spent a lot of money on her dress, and we also paid for the bridesmaids' outfits. Her younger sister, Mandy, was the maid of honour, and I was quite close to her. She had a very kind nature, and she was an intelligent, pretty girl, and had I been single, I would have pursued her. But I am not a cheat – I had not cheated for twelve years and was not about to start with Mandy. Hailey's family were all kind to me and often told me they knew what she was like and that they always had my back.

Hailey had an older sister, Gail, who was a fun woman, maybe ten years older than me. She often babysat for us so we could go out for meals and let our hair down. One evening during a fun night out with the family at a Chinese restaurant with an Elvis impersonator, we all got very, very drunk. Gail was gay and had a lovely girlfriend, but she had a soft spot for me. And during our meal, she was very, very drunk and now and then lifted her top and bra, flashing me her boobs. I had no feeling for her in that way, but I loved her fun nature and I laughed so much that night. If ever you get the chance to see a Chinese Elvis impersonator in a Chinese restaurant, I urge you to go.

The morning of the wedding, I stayed at Gail's house, and as I stood in front a full-length mirror doing up my cravat, I popped two Diazepam I'd been given by her to calm my frayed nerves. I looked at myself and said, I do not want to do this. I never did, but I was doing it for my son, Daniel. I never told him it was the only reason I had married his mother and am unsure what he would think, but I felt it was the 'right' thing to do by him.

As friends and family turned up before the ceremony, I mingled. Hailey had warned me to not have a single drink at the pub opposite the church where we all met, and even with that, I still walked in and married her, for better or for worse. . . . It got worse, for richer or poorer. I ended up much poorer, in sickness and health. After the ceremony, we went to our reception in a small hall in Sidcup with a decent disco, nice food, and £500 behind the bar. We had a video booth for our guests to leave us messages of goodwill. The next day, we flew off to Lanzarote on our honeymoon. We consummated our marriage once on our honeymoon and once only. The only joy I experienced over that trip was from the crazy group of Germans in the bar every night, grabbing hold of me and getting me drunk and dancing with them. They spoke no English, and I spoke no German, but it was so much fun.

On our return, I was moved to a different branch of the sofa company in Sidcup. The staff were not as friendly; in fact, there were quite a few nasty arseholes working there. I got on well with two of the girls in the office: one I fancied, but she was seeing a guy in the warehouse, so I had no chance; and the other girl who looked after service was cute but was just a friend. And I would never cheat, regardless. By this time, I recruited one of my old staff from my previous job, a lovely girl named Ann. My manager at Sidcup was the most miserable, sanctimonious bastard you could ever want to work for. He led by fear and dread, so we clashed. Hailey phoned me a lot at work, and it did me no favours. I was called over by the area manager (the guy who had recruited me) and he told me I could either leave or he would force me out. He told me there were several reasons for this, one being the number of phone calls I got at work, which I accepted. Then he began making shit up, like I was always late. When I tried to tell him that I was, in fact, always thirty minutes early so I could grab a coffee and have a smoke, he shut me down. He did that with a few other things that were also untrue. If he had said to me, Darren, the phone calls have to stop, or I will let you go, I would have agreed. But the other shit was not fair.

I called up another local furniture store and spoke to the manager, who seemed pleasant. Before long, I was working for them. If I thought the popular sofa store was cliquey, they had nothing on the furniture store. If you did not fit in, you were out. I was okay with the manageress, although she could be very neurotic, like the time I was mopping the toilet floor and she came in screaming in a full rage that I was missing parts. I could have cried and punched her in the face both at the same time. There were also some genuine characters in the store, like the deputy manager, who was a slimeball arse-licker; the hard man who thought he was the bee's knees; the wet drip who sold beds; the polite, well-educated, and very well-dressed middle-aged woman; a Scouser who could make anyone cry with laughter within two minutes of talking to him; and then my dear friend Alan (RIP). I would pop upstairs and chat to Alan now and then. He was about sixty-four years old and always had a tale to tell. One day I told him my grandfather was a Freemason, and a little twinkle in his eye appeared. He told me he was, too, and in fact, he was the master of his lodge. Over six months, we talked about Freemasonry, and they invited me to apply. After couple of interviews and some background checks, I was invited into Alan's lodge. It was an enormous honour and something I had wanted to do ever since I was a little boy. I would often ask my grandad to shake my hand and try to guess what the secret was. He would just laugh and laugh at me.

After work, it was common for the manager to pass around a few beers, and we would chat for forty minutes before heading home. One night, I mentioned that I had been given some brand-new white Calvin Klein boxers and shorts that were small and I was large. They asked me how much I wanted for them and if they were boxed. The next day, I brought them in and the Scouser offered to buy them. I realised when I picked them up from home that they were not boxed but didn't think it would be a problem. I pulled them out in front of the entire team of maybe ten of us, and he took them from me to check the size. As he opened them up, he looked inside and, to my horror, told me there was a huge skid mark on one of the pants. I was so embarrassed as he showed all the staff, telling them I was trying to sell second-hand skiddy underpants for five pounds. I threw the pants in my bottom drawer and forgot about them, but now and then, the story came up that at least they didn't sell shitty underpants to workmates for a fiver. Six months later, my manager had cause to go through my drawers and found my drawers, and I got a huge bollocking and was asked to please take my soiled underpants home.

The furniture store also owned a bed shop in Bromley, and a young guy who was a bit of a boy around town ran it. Occasionally, we would be asked to go over and help for the day. Scouser seemed to enjoy it, so he spent a lot of time in the store. One morning, I went to find them both asleep on two of the new beds, still dressed, stinking of booze, and one of them had puked on the showroom bed. I was horrified and did not go back to the store again. A few weeks later, we heard that the two of them had been asking for cash for the beds that were sold and, instead of banking it, were going out on the town and spending the money on champagne and cocktails, then crashing on the beds in the store. Word got out, and they both disappeared. The store called in the police, and they figured out that an enormous amount of money had been taken. Last I heard, the Scouser was working on the dustcarts.

Our manager was offered a larger store in Croydon and we had a new manager come in. He was my age and oozed smarm. At every opportunity, this smart aleck would haul me over the coals in his office, berating me for anything and everything. I guess my face did not fit. One day, I saw two young guys carrying an expensive coffee table out of the front door. I thought this was odd, as we did not sell stock; we ordered it. I followed them out and asked them for their receipt, but they kept walking, just ignoring me. They put it into a false-plated old Fiesta, and I began punching the side window to no avail and screaming at them. We called the police, but they did nothing.

That time came again where I was asked to leave, and with a heavy heart, I began looking around once more.

Chapter Twenty-Two
Pitney Bowes

One of Hailey's sisters worked in a spa and massage centre. But Hailey would have none of it and went around telling everyone her sister was a prostitute. The shit hit the fan, and one night, at 11:00 p.m., we had her and her stepmom banging on our door, yelling abuse. To be fair, I couldn't blame them, and that then sparked a family feud, one of many. Why you would tell everyone such a thing, even if it was true, was beyond my comprehension. She was so hateful and aggressive for no reason. When Hailey had been born, her mum was taking a lot of drugs and could not cope, so Hailey was brought up by her stepmom, Margaret. Her mother, Denise, met another man, and she had a second daughter, Mandy. The same thing happened, and their stepmom, Margaret, took care of them both. Hailey always felt that she was thrown away by her mother and that her stepmother had kidnapped her, but this could not have been further from the truth. Mandy knew the truth and never twisted it, but Hailey had issues with abandonment and could never find the love she felt she needed. She also trusted no one . . . which is why she struggled with relationships so much and earned her nickname at the sofa store, 'Psycho'. When Hailey and Mandy found out their true parentage, they also found out that their older sisters were their aunties by blood. But it changed nothing; they still loved them both.

They all knew I had issues. You could be sure Hailey had told them that and would milk it for all its worth for sympathy. Oh, Darren is having another episode . . . poor me. I am not saying I did not have terrible spells, but I was really more stable than her.

I had worked with a guy at Computer Land that was now a headhunter for a recruitment company. He had kept in contact, and every few months, we would chat about what jobs were knocking around. I called him, and he told me about a job that would be right up my street: selling franking machines. I gasped when he mentioned them, and as a seasoned salesperson, I knew you have to believe in your product. How could I get passionate about putting a stamp mark on an envelope? The company, Pitney Bowes, was a huge American business that had the franking machine market tied up in the US and the UK. I was told that there would be a three-stage interview process, and it was difficult. He told me that at the last stage, even if they wanted you, occasionally they would say no and that it would be down to you not to accept no and demand the job, just like you would when knocked back in the field when selling. They did not want salespeople who were not hungry and let sales slip through their hands. I only remember one interview and it was with the area manager, Sean, and manager, Dave. I was given a random pen and asked to sell it to them. Being a smart-ass, I decided that a crappy £20 pen was not worthy of these fine sales executives and tried to upsell them a PDA, which was worth much more. A PDA was a small tablet-like gadget you wrote on. Why would they want to walk into a meeting for an enormous deal with a plastic pen when they could walk in with the latest tech? I was unsure what they thought, but I was told afterwards I sold the pen, and I argued that in the real world I would have upsold them. I remember having to do a presentation on a paper board which went well, and the pressure was quite intense.

I got the job and started two weeks later. I was told I would have to attend a two-week residential course at a hotel, and Hailey flipped her lid that I would be away with other women in a hotel. We argued about me taking the job, but it gave a nice brand-new Ford Focus, £34K a year with commission paid on top, and was a step upwards. There were about twenty-two of us at the course and the atmosphere was great. We had lectures during the day on selling techniques, hands-on practice with the machines, and how to generate our own leads in the patches field they gave us. At the end of the two weeks, we were tested, and it was a case of pass, you are in; fail, you are out . . . so not much pressure, then. I started in our London office, but we soon moved to Surrey, which is why they had taken on so many new employees. The new office was quite large and much nicer than our old one. They gave me my area, Kent, a large county to the southeast of London, which was a vast area to cover. I spent Tuesday to Friday driving to offices and industrial parks and trying to get a card from each business with the name of the managing director and telephone number. The receptionists were inundated with sales reps barging in trying to contact the MD and had become successful MD gatekeepers. All week, we collected cards, and took notes about the companies – for instance, did they have a franking machine; if so, which one; etc. On the Monday after, we would all go into the Redhill office and spend the day on the phones trying our damnedest to get hold of the MDs and then make an appointment to talk to them about all the delights of franking machines. I would arrange all cold-canvassing appointments. Once in with the managing director, we had to sell the idea of what a franking machine would do for the possible prestige of the company, such as a printed company logo next to the frank, and how it was so much more professional than licking a stamp, and you never ran out like you did with stamps. It was also far more time-efficient when posting, as they slid through the machine quickly. The catch, though, was that not only did they have to pay the same for the postage which would be digital – they also had to contract hire the machine. Sales were rare – like unicorn shit rare – and I only ever sold a few in my time there.

Just before Christmas, we were told we had to attend a pub crawl around London, but I had a two-year-old toddler and a paranoid, neurotic wife, so I declined. My area manager, Sean, told me it was not something I could turn down, and so I met everyone in Covent Garden. With about twenty-five of us crammed into a dingy bar, the rounds began flooding in. We all bought a double tequila, and I turned it down, knowing what would happen if I chugged it. They would have none of it, and so I warned them to move out of the way. They didn't take my request seriously at all, and so I threw it down my throat. Within about five seconds, I was projectile vomiting all over the bar's floor to the screams of horror from my colleagues. 'I tried to bloody warn you', I told them, laughing.

'Yup, but why didn't you at least try to run to the toilet?' they asked me.

That would be known for the rest of my time at the company as 'the tequila incident'.

As the evening progressed, a couple of us went to Chinatown for some munch. As we were walking down the street, we bumped into Sean and he joined us. We were eating our food and started talking about how we were going to get home, as the trains stopped at 10:45 p.m. I was very fortunate to have a friend whom I called and offered £30 to come collect us. Sean was over the moon, as was my other colleague, and I think it stood me in good stead.

Our small team was led by our manager, a dapper young guy named Dave. He was a nice guy, hungry for us to succeed, and came out occasionally to see how we were doing. I remember meeting up with him in a Tesco car park one day whilst out on the road. My car was strewn with paperwork all over the seat, and he was horrified. I felt awful, as I did not want to disappoint him and he was mentoring us, too. As time went on, I got friendly with two girls on my team. I will admit to fancying Veronica, but she had a boyfriend in the company and her father was the UK manager. I would never cheat, and in all fairness, I don't think there was any attraction, but she was pleasant company, and when bored, I would call her whilst pounding the industrial estates of Kent.

Hailey often went through my mobile phone and towards the end began calling and texting the two girls, warning them away from me. It was so embarrassing. But they were amazing about it. Hailey was becoming worse at home, and we were spending a fortune on our house. She wanted the best of everything, and because I was working, all the finance went in my name. We had a brand-new fitted kitchen with real stone tiles on the floor and walls. We had a Schreiber-fitted bedroom with fitted wardrobes and a bridge over the bed, a plush royal-blue carpet, and during my time at the sofa company, we had bought a super king-size Vispring bed. It cost £7,500, but I got a staff discount and it was a beast of a bed. It said, I am obsessed with sleep or/and sex, which is quite ironic because during our nine months of marriage, we only had sex three or four times. Next to our bedroom was a spare room leading down from the side of my room. We didn't need it as a bedroom, so we made a huge en suite. Hailey's brother was a self-employed plumber, and we asked him to do the work for us. We had a large vanity unit and a two-man jacuzzi corner bath. It looked outstanding, and her brother did a cracking job. When we asked him how much we owed him, we were surprised that he charged us full price. When queried, he told us that had he spent the week elsewhere, he would have gotten the same money. I always felt he could have knocked a bit off and that he was mean for doing that.

Things were shaking at the seams for Hailey and me. She was so verbally and mentally abusive to me, and so much shouting and screaming in the house made me unhappy. She turned me away from my family, who would always tell me to leave her. They had said right from the beginning that she was a nutcase. I had chatted to an old friend from years ago, Mitch – the same guy who had dated Hazel back in Shoe Express. It was his birthday, and he wanted me to go out with him and his friends. They were going to Spearmint Rhino in London, which was a very fancy, upmarket strip club. Hailey spat her dummy out and would not let me go. Eventually, I snapped and walked out. It was not even about going to a strip club for me; it was about her control. I stayed at Mitch's for a few days, and she was on the phone crying. I went to see her, and she explained the reason she had not wanted sex was because she had been sexually abused. I cannot confirm this, as she was always so full of lies, but she promised to go to counselling for her issues, and so I agreed to work things out with her. Later that night, we had sex. A few days later, though, the screaming started again. I don't think she could control it, and I realised she would never change. I had been foolish to believe she could. I was right to leave the first time. And so, I walked out a second time, but this time I never went back. I sofa surfed for a couple of months and things were awful for me.

One day whilst I was on the road, Hailey phoned me and she was having sex with someone, screaming, and moaning down the phone. I was distraught that she could be so evil and callous, but there was much worse to come. I was struggling financially and had not opened up a separate account yet. I went to my nan, cap in hand, and asked to borrow £500 to tide me over. I'll never forget her asking, 'Will Hailey get hold of this?', and I reassured her Hailey would not know. The next day I went to withdraw the £500 to keep me going to find out Hailey had taken it that morning. I called her and she just laughed. I cried so hard that afternoon that I had to cancel my appointments. I sat outside my appointment sobbing and sobbing, and then had to tell my nan what Hailey had done. I felt so awful.

I stayed at my mum's bungalow in Hazelmere and received another call from Hailey. As the phone rang, I felt sick to the bottom of my stomach. Whenever she called, it was never good. 'I have something to tell you, Darren,' she said. 'I am pregnant, hahaha.'

And then she put the phone down. I cried again and again at how evil, twisted, and manipulative she was. I wrung my hands in my mum's kitchen as I told her I just could not cope and life was so awful and dark. She comforted me and told me to get a solicitor.

Chapter Twenty-Three
Site Work

My mum and nan both lived in Hazelmere in Surrey, so it meant a long commute to Kent every day. I slept on a Z bed in my nan's dining room and it was hard going. I was happy at Pitney Bowes, but I was becoming quite tired in myself. One salesperson there had been a CPN in his former job. He told me he had left because the money was so much better here and his old job was way too stressful. I told him of my diagnosis and that I was struggling, and all he could say was 'See your local CMHT', so I did.

One day, Sean approached me and told me he would like to come out with me for the day and we pencilled it in. I told him I had a few good leads and that I would book them all in for the day together. Sean and I set out for our first appointment, and they signed up. I was overjoyed, and so was Sean. They were the first sales I had made in six months, and when we got back to the office, Sean could not sing my praises highly enough and told the other staff I was an animal, and I felt so chuffed. Payday came, and they gave me a bottle of champagne and a hefty bonus.

Although my work life was flourishing, my home life was hell on earth. Christmas was approaching, and I wanted to see my eldest, Daniel, and my new-born son, Joshua. Hailey said no and I spoke to my solicitor, who wrote to hers, begging for me to see them. I later realised the solicitors were fleecing me, just sending endless letters at £35 a pop, and the whole thing cost me £2,300 and I maxed my credit card. I got rid of these solicitors, as they just used people to cash in.

At the time, during 2002, I decided I had had enough of everything and handed my notice in. I needed time to recuperate. I lost my company car, but I had a large motorbike, a Yamaha YZF750R, which was an absolute beast and became my only method of transport. My uncle, Barry, owned a medium-sized construction company, and I went to work for him, labouring. I think I earned about £900 a month and the work was hard. The first day, I had to litter pick a warehouse, which was the size of two football pitches, and my back was breaking. The jarring pain throbbed up my back, and I felt I would fall over, but I just kept going. Soon, I got used to the work and much fitter. One day, they offered me a job to paint three piles of five hundred twenty-foot wooden slats and told me I would get £250 for painting them. My uncle figured it would take me three or four days to do one lot of five hundred. I asked around and got a friend and another guy. I told them we had to knock it out in one day and it would be hard work. I paid them £100 cash in hand, which at the time was fair money. It was a hard day's graft. Word got out to my uncle that I had finished them and hired guys and that he owed me £750 for a day's work. To say he was furious was an understatement. Saying that the whole construction industry is all about contracting work out, he could say nothing, and I made £550 in one day. After chatting to a few of the workers, they told me that qualified plumbers were earning crazy money, but it had been years since I had been on the tools and could not just walk into a job with no tools and no experience for eight years. After some research, my uncle told me about a local company that did simple maintenance work. They supplied a van and tools, so it was a sure thing as long as I could get a job there.

I spoke to the boss and arranged an interview. I turned up on my motorbike and he told me he, too, was a biker, and that sealed the deal. The day I started, I was given a van and taken down to the local tool shop with one supervisor. He walked around, picking up everything I needed. I was like a kid at Christmas in a toy shop. Most of the work was going out on my own and doing minor jobs like fixing faulty boilers in pubs we had contracts with. Anything I was unsure about, I just called in for advice. They did some site work in a gang of four or five, but it was piss-simple work, if dull. Nevertheless, I was gaining the ever-needed experience and building up my own tools.

During this time, I received a phone call from a writer from Chat Magazine. Chat Magazine was a young woman's trashy mag with vile sensational stories. She told me she was writing Hailey's story about how she'd lived with a schizophrenic and how I had walked out, leaving her in mountains of debt. I begged her not to print it, as it would ruin my reputation and was nobody's business but mine. I spent weeks worried sick about the story and if people I knew, including my employer, would see it and manage me out. The magazine was published, and I was featured on the front page – 'Oh Lord, my husband is God again' – with a picture. I read the article and it showed Hailey with the kids and the biggest pile of shit stories. The only decent thing was the fact they printed some decent photos of me. I was distraught, and they paid her £500 for telling my story. I will never forgive her for that.

In all fairness, the plumbing company was quite nice to work for, but I had my sights set on doing self-employed on-site work on new houses. I paid for the ACS gas safety course and spent Saturdays studying before finally sitting the exam. The course was very expensive at £2,500, but meant I could fit boilers, cookers, and meters on-site, which was rare and commanded top dollar. I spoke to the maintenance company and told them I was leaving, and they offered me an extra £2,000 to stay, but

£24,000 could not compare with being self-employed, so I said my goodbyes.

I found work easily, and during my phone call with the owner, he asked about my experience and he asked how much I wanted a day. I told him £200 a day for day work, and I soon started. There was some price work, but one of his mates worked on-site and had that sewn up, throwing plastic pipework in for radiators. It was child's play and paid very well. I was asked to fit unvented heating and hot water systems, which were complicated, and I'd never done one, so I copied one that had already been done and was fine. For some odd reason, the boss began pouring responsibility onto me like I was a foreman and asking me why the site was not progressing faster. I felt like telling him I was not a paid foreman, even if I was qualified. He didn't appreciate it and he began moving me around sites and finishing fuck-ups from his mate. I had to commission one particular house, and when I turned the water on, I realised his mate had connected the powerful mains to the plastic radiator pipework, and it blew every single radiator valve off every radiator. The house flooded, and I was so fucked off with his shoddy work. I complained, but I got the blame for not checking. He had crossed over his pipework, and I realised they were fuckwits. Another time we had to get the show house ready, and the deadline was two days. His fuckwit mate and I commissioned it, and one of the plastic flows and return pipes blew a joint in the ceiling – and the kitchen flooded. We had to cut the ceiling to repair it and the boss went ape shit, as did the site supervisor. I don't know why they got shitty with me. I had done no work inside at all. They kept all of our materials in one garage and I held the keys. But once a week, his fuckwit mate would pull out piles of new copper pipe and fitting, telling me he sold them at car boot sales. I was so angry at him for doing this to his mate but felt little sympathy for the boss, as he backed everything the fuckwit did every time, so I said nothing. Taking a few bits to do a minor job at home was fair game, but fuckwit had thousands. He was also stealing red diesel from the site, which was used for machinery like digger trucks. He did not pay for any diesel, but using red diesel in a road vehicle was a very serious offence, as it was so cheap and no tax or duty was paid on it, even if he was stealing it. Every week, he pumped the barrels into jerry cans. He was a weasel.

One Saturday, I sat in the tea room and the site work supervisor sat reading the Star newspaper, and I had been warned that my Chat Magazine story was featured within it that particular day. It was in the magazine and he read it. Nothing was said, but I was told on Monday that he wanted me off-site. Complete discrimination, right there in black-and-white. I had had enough by that time, so I left. I went to collect my weekly cheque of £750 only to be told they were knocking me. I was furious, but also helpless. But karma came to my rescue, as a week later, I had a call to ask if I still had the keys to the lockup. Yes, of course I did, and they were not getting them back until I was paid. I made sure I was paid, and the cheque cleared, and then handed back the keys.

Since leaving Hailey, I had tried to socialise with friends. I began knocking around with Hazel's old boyfriend, Mitch. He lived in a nice small house in Leatherhead with his girlfriend, Sally, and a mate named Gary. Both of them had picked up the motorcycle bug, and both passed their tests. We hung out with another friend, Rob, and spent hours riding around. At the time, I had a Yamaha YZF750R, and it was way too big for me. It was so heavy and I dropped it twice on diesel in a petrol station. I was living in Hazelmere in Surrey, so it would take me an hour to get to Mitch's in Leatherhead. We went out every Friday and Saturday night, pubbing and clubbing, and tore around the roads like nutcases. There were a few parties and I met a couple of girls, but in all honesty, I hated women after all my terrible experiences. I met a girl one night in a local pub and after a cheeky snog, she asked if I wanted to go back for the night and I said no. She copped the strop and called me a cock tease, but I just wasn't interested in anyone. I had a couple of admirers, too, but I brushed them off. I heard from Hailey once or twice, but it was usually bad news. She had been told by staff at DFS that I'd had an affair with one of the girls I liked. Chance would have been a fine thing, but I found it funny the girl lied about being with me and wished I had gotten her number.

I had long thought about Sue, and had a lot of ghosts I wanted to put to bed, so I plucked up the courage to write to her at her old address. I cannot remember what I wrote, but within a week, I got a call on my mobile from her. I was at Mitch's house. It was a Saturday morning, and it shocked me when she called. She asked if she could meet me, and I told her I was at a friend's house in Leatherhead. Shocked, she asked me where, as she lived in a Leatherhead herself. When I told her, she said she lived on the same road and was a two-minute walk away. Sue knocked on the door fifteen minutes later and I gave her a hug, and she was so excited to see me. She looked well, although slimmer than she had been years ago. She presented herself immaculately. We caught up with light chitchat, and she told me she had moved in with Andrew from university, but that they only lasted a couple of years. Sue had then married her now-husband, but he was violent towards her and I'm sure she was quite unhappy. She was still a wild child, and I think she still smoked the wacky back and did a lot of photoshoots with her sexy figure and pretty face. We decided that we would catch up soon and talk about old times.

Chapter Twenty-Four
Sam

That night we had gone to Chicago Rock Cafe in Sutton, a bar/disco that played eighties music. It was the place you go to at the end of the night when the pubs closed, got even drunker, had a dance, and tried to grab a snog. I never was one for taking girls home – not my style. I was happy with a kiss and a number. But this night was going to be very different. Gary and I had trawled the pubs in Sutton and ended up at Chicago's. They rammed the club full of revellers dancing, drinking, and having fun. I got two pints of lager at the bar, which I struggled to carry back to our little spot by the top of the venue. I looked around and could not see Gary anywhere, so I stood there, looking like a lost sheep. A voice piped up next to me saying, 'He's in the toilet.' I looked over in my drunken state and saw a pretty girl sitting in a wheelchair. I thanked her and she wheeled herself back to her group of friends not far away. Gary came back, and I told him I'd seen a lovely girl. And with no tact at all, he turned 180 degrees and stared at her, making it obvious I had asked him to check her out. Embarrassed, we went over and began chatting to the group. There were three of them in total. We chatted and took turns to buy rounds, which was not the done thing. The done thing was for the guys to buy all the drinks, hoping to get lucky – I didn't feel lucky. I asked the girl's name, and she told me it was Sam. I was very drunk, but I could tell she was slim and pretty with shoulder-length brown hair. I asked her friend if she liked me, and I told her I wanted to kiss her.

Her friend said, 'Go on, then.'

I did.

One of Sam's friends was a nice-looking girl who fancied Gary, but he stayed away. I had never known him to have a girlfriend or boyfriend but never questioned his sexuality; he was a friend, and it did not matter. At the end of the night, I asked Sam for her mobile number and promised to call or text her. I texted her over the next couple of days and then called her, asking if she would like to meet up for a date. She said yes and asked me over to her flat on Wednesday evening in Wallington just outside of Croydon.

I turned up at 8:00 p.m. and knocked on the door. A minute later, the door opened, and I caught sight of her. I was absolutely blown away. Sam was stunning, and in an instant, I fell in love and knew at that moment I wanted to spend the rest of my life with her. She was wearing a mustard top with small flowers; her hair was a rich dark auburn with blonde highlights. She was wearing makeup and had a smile that made me go weak at the knees. Her dark sculpted brows accentuated her deep-blue eyes. Sam had a firm jaw and her hair cupped it gently. She was tall, even though she was sitting. She had beautiful broad shoulders and strong biceps where she would propel her chair. The rest of her was slim and toned. We went through to the lounge, and she transferred herself to her sofa; I sat next to her, and we chatted and enjoyed loving kisses and cuddles. I found it so easy to talk to Sam, and my old guard came down as she held my heart in her hand. I visited her every night, and we texted when we were not together. In short, I was smitten. On Saturday night, I stayed over, and we made love, and I never went home. Sam would later tell me she had arrived at Chicago's at 11:30 p.m., and as she came up the ramp, she'd seen me and something inside her had made her think she had to talk to me. So, when Gary had gone to the toilet later, she'd grabbed her opportunity.

Sam soon told me she had Friedreich's ataxia, which is an incredibly rare terminal degenerative neurological condition that affects one in every fifty thousand people. It can cause early death in some, mostly with issues affecting the heart, but people can go on to live long lives just like Sam. She could not walk, as she had muscle wastage in her legs, and she suffered with spasticity, causing her arms and legs to painfully spasm.

Chapter Twenty-Five
Wallington

The first few weeks with Sam were a whirlwind. I was staying every night, and over two weeks, I began slowly moving more things in until a month later, I was fully moved in. In fact, I felt so serious about Sam that two weeks after we met, I took her to meet my mum and we had a Sunday roast dinner. When I was in the kitchen, Mum pulled me to one side and told me sternly to not break Sam's heart, and I told her I would not. We sat around the dinner table, and being in her chair eating at the table was difficult, but it was one of many challenges we would face together.

Sam's home was a large, converted house. She had downstairs as a flat, and her parents had upstairs as a flat. The idea was to give someone with a disability independence but with family close for support. Sam had an amazing life. She would go to a club for disabled people during the day where they would do crafts, have lunch, and chat. At night, she was out with her many friends, getting drunk and enjoying her life. She did work with her family, who owned a dry cleaner's shop, and at one time they had had a gift shop above it. Sam had wanted to go to university when she was younger, but we did not have the support back in the day for people who needed extra help. The flat was spacious, with a huge lounge with lovely bay windows, a long kitchen, a double bedroom, and a nice wet room bathroom. There was a small patio garden out the back where we could sit and have a coffee. Over the years, we decorated and modernised the furniture and fittings together.

During the time we met, Sam's mum was in Australia and had come back early, but because her mum had been told Sam had met someone, she did not let Sam know she was home. Every time I drove out to work, they would peek through the windows to catch a glimpse of me. Finally, her mum came down and I sat on the sofa, nervous but excited to meet her. Julie was a lot younger than my mum. She was friendly and yet incredibly blunt, which took some getting used to because I hate being confrontational. A spade was a spade with Julie, and if you didn't like it, you could fuck off. Sam's dad was a lovely man named Ron who owned his own dry cleaner business close by in a little town called Ashtead, and they were both hard workers. Sam had two brothers: Dave was younger than Sam, and he worked in the family business; Jay was a teenager who did not work. Shortly after Sam and I met, Dave met his current wife, Amy, and they are still together eighteen years later with two sons.

At the time, site work was getting tedious and I was becoming frustrated, so I looked around for something different. I found a job fitting solar-heated hot water cylinders. There was a three-day training period, and then I shadowed a fellow fitter for a week before being given my work. The company was based in Chelmsford, which was a fair drive once a week to pick up all the materials. The job was very demanding but paid well, although I was on the road at 6:30 a.m. and not in most nights until 8:30. The job consisted of changing the hot water cylinder for a designed new one and connecting it to a solar collecting panel on the roof and wiring the system up and commissioning it. The work required hard and long hours and within six months, I was pretty burnt out. A lot of plumbers did not last in the job, so there was a large turnover. The company charged £7.5K, and the work took about two to three days from my end, and a day or two for the roofer to fit the panels, so they were making money hand over fist. I felt their sales staff were sharp selling, as they told customers that light was enough to heat the water but, in fact, it needed sunshine, and it did not sit well with me. I can say I have never met so many obnoxious customers in all my time. They all seemed angry and pushy, even whilst I tried to be polite.

Sam and I got on great and I felt so happy. My sister Jennine had two children, Laura, and William, of a similar age to my two, and it was lovely seeing them with my kids. We babysat for them during holidays, and they would come over to our flat in Wallington and Sam would do things like making candles with them or baking cakes. I would teach them how to play *World of Warcraft*, and we had a great time killing boars and spiders with their little gnome characters.

We lost touch with most of our friends, which was both of our faults. It happens to many new couples, but I regret Sam losing hers. As for Mitch and Gary, something happened that made me bitter for a long time. During a visit to my mum's one day, Mitch called me and was on loudspeaker on my mobile. He asked me what colour Sam's knickers were; I was bouncing and in no uncertain terms told him to fuck off. 'No worries,' he said, 'I'll ask her when I see her on Saturday.' From that moment onwards, I stopped trusting friends, which was sad for me. For my best mate to do that broke my heart, and I felt I could no longer trust any male friend. Sue kept in touch and would call me now and then. She wrote me a couple of letters, too, and one told me I was still as handsome as I'd been when we were together. I did not realise just how hurtful this was to Sam, and it seemed Sue might still have feelings for me. For me, Sue was just a friend, but I told her I could no longer keep in contact. Sue told me Sam had nothing to fear from her, but I could not let Sam suffer, so I said goodbye.

One afternoon in 2006, Sam got a severe pain in her leg. We called our local GP out for a home visit and she spent around ten days on the sofa with me rubbing creams into them to no avail. After ten days, she got a pain in her chest. The GP was head of his practice, an elderly man, and told Sam he could not detect any DVT or blood clot in her leg, and if it got worse to visit accident and emergency. The next day, I was unhappy with her condition and drove her down. The register took a blood test and put her on an ECG machine and told us straight that it was near enough guaranteed she had a blood clot on her lung. They took her up to the ward and she was put on a vast amount of morphine and heparin injections, as she was in agony. It was a scary time and Sam was so drugged up, she began hallucinating, hearing and seeing awful things. She was also being sick every fifteen minutes, and they left it down to me to sit her forward, as she could not do it herself, to vomit into a cardboard container. I was cross that the nurses did not offer to sit with her.

She was delirious and screaming that her mum was stuck under the bed and they were coming to get her. It was awful. She was in the ward for about twelve days and in a bad way when her consultant visited her and immediately told them to get her off the morphine or she would leave via the morgue. Thankfully, she got better and finally came home. And according to the staff, she cheated death, albeit she would forever be on blood thinners.

After coming out of the hospital, Sam's health deteriorated drastically. She could no longer transfer herself into and out of her wheelchair, cook, or dress anymore, so we decided I would give up work and care for her full-time. The transition was painful financially. I visited the same GP myself during a period of paranoia and he asked me, 'Who is after you this time – Noddy?' I was shell-shocked that a senior doctor could be so blasé and rude about a serious mental health symptom. Paranoia is one of the worst symptoms of schizophrenia – feeling like you are being watched, filmed, and monitored is petrifying, and for him to belittle me like that was unforgivable. After both of our incidents, we changed doctors to a new larger surgery in town, and they were much better.

My mental health had been very up and down over the years. I had periods where I felt I was being watched and followed. I also suffered from the negative symptoms of lethargy and lack of motivation. When we were out and about in Wallington High Street, I would tell Sam I felt paranoid and that it was overwhelming. She would hug me and reassure me I was safe and nobody would hurt me. Sam gave me the courage to be more open about my fears.

Chapter Twenty-Six
Money

I claimed government benefits which, compared to my £38K a year, could not have been more shocking. I was smoking three packets of cigarettes a day, which were not cheap, and I was used to a certain lifestyle. The biggest problem for me was the vast amount of debt I was in after leaving Hailey. I owed £24K, and the vast majority of that was from luxuries at my old marital home. None of the finance was in Hailey's name, which was quite cunning of her. I asked her to sell our house, which had a fair amount of collateral, or buy me out. I did not want half; I just wanted what I had put in, which ironically was the same as the debt. She declined, so I went to a solicitor who begged her to buy me out; otherwise, I would have no other option but to go bankrupt. I was getting daily phone calls from collection agencies and it was a stressful time. Not seeing my sons just made this all even worse. My mental health was waning because of the ongoing stress. I was still hearing voices and had slight paranoia. I regularly saw a CPN in the Sutton CMHT.

Hailey refused to budge on our house, so whilst I went ahead with our divorce, I also filed for bankruptcy. It was a horrible experience walking into court and handing over £350 cash and standing in front of a judge to explain my situation. I was released six months later, but being bankrupt meant I could not get credit for six months and was only allowed a basic bank account with a debit card. Everything was written off, barring my student loan which, being from the government, was exempt. Hailey's solicitor began freaking out via letters that I would put our house at risk by going bankrupt. I do not know why or how they didn't realise I would have to do this, as we had written to them at least three or four times, explaining I had no option unless I was paid out only the deposit I had put in, not the £100K equity that was tied up. I was happy for her to keep it all; I just wanted to be debt-free. Eventually, my creditors would go after it and force a sale, but it took ten years. Hailey got legal aid, which I did not, and so she tried every trick in the book and lied to keep it, from our children's health to her not being told when we'd bought our home that it would be in joint names, even though it had been explained to her twice. Why would she lie and think anyone would believe she would be the sole owner when we'd bought it just before we were married? She accused her solicitor and his PA of not telling us. I remembered the conversation and the PA's name, so it did not get her anywhere. The main issue I had after ten years of legal wrangling with her barristers meant all of my share that was leftover was eaten up in legal fees. I got nothing. And she did get something. Not only did I not see my children, but I'd lost my five-bedroom home and had gone bankrupt. But at least I had my lovely Sam, and she kept me fighting. It was not long before Hailey was up to her nasty tricks again, and we had a huge argument on the phone. She told me that unless I saw the kids three times a month, I would be banned from seeing them. I was so upset and angry that Hailey would use my own children as a weapon against me but accepted that when they were old enough, they would come looking for me. A part of me died that day.

Sam's parents owned a static caravan in West Wales in a lovely county called Carmarthenshire. We would go up twice a year for a brief break and would spend most of our time sitting around, drinking coffee.

Our favourite place we used to call our own was a lovely seaside town called Saundersfoot. It was on the west coast of Wales, close to Tenby, and it had a lovely long sandy beach. We would sit on the beachfront with a bag of chips and gravy and either read or people watch. There was a lovely shop that sold sweets of all kinds, and we would walk out with candy floss or clotted cream fudge. It was a bubbly town where families bustled around, with old couples walking hand in hand. I had never seen such massive seagulls in my life, and they were all waiting to pounce on a dropped chip.

One evening, we went to the site's club and sat, having a beer, when the conversation turned to marriage. I had always said after Hailey that I would never marry again, and Sam had always said she never wanted to marry. But that night, I turned to Sam and told her I would marry her, and she said that she felt the same way. We had only been together for maybe eight months, and Hailey was dragging her heels with the divorce, so I began the proceedings myself. A week after coming back from the caravan, Sam and I were lying on our lounge floor on a duvet, eating pizza and chatting. She brought up our conversation, and then asked, 'Should we do it?'

I asked her, 'Do what?' She called me a fool and told me about getting married. I turned and told her, 'Yeah, okay', and grinned at her. We were engaged for a long time, maybe two and a half years. When we began planning our wedding, Sam's mum began getting a bit carried away and suggesting this and that, and it was things we didn't want. I can't blame her, as Sam had never thought she would marry, so her mum was excited. We tried to quell the enthusiasm, but it didn't work, so we cancelled everything. About a month later, we set a new date and told everyone we were arranging everything and to leave it to us. We had little money, being on benefits, and we just wanted a small wedding. We picked Sutton Registry Office which, in all fairness, was lovely.

The morning of the wedding, I saw Sam in her dress. Her wheelchair had been decorated with ribbons and she looked divine. We only had immediate family plus one of my oldest friends, Hazel, as my best man, otherwise known as the best bird. Sam's uncle had flown over from Australia, and bless him, he videoed everything. We did not have a photographer, so my dad took plenty of pictures. On 8 September 2006, we took our vows in the registry office, repeating the words read out to us by the clerk: 'I do lawfully take . . .' Mischievously, I said, 'I do awfully take Samantha', which got a few giggles. Hazel read a poem during the service. Somebody took a picture of her, and it is the nicest picture I have of her. Afterwards, we had photographs taken in the lovely back garden of the office. We drove home to our flat in Wallington and my sister Melanie had made a lovely pink wedding cake with a beautiful bow around it. We had a few drinks, and people relaxed and chatted until the evening when we all went down to our favourite restaurant, the Shanghai Chinese restaurant. The owner had set up a large area for us with all the tables together. We sat and ate a delicious Chinese meal for our wedding, and it was glorious. My best bird Hazel did herself proud and embarrassed the hell out of me during her speech.

The next day, we drove up to the caravan for a week in sunny Wales, but it rained every day and we came home after five days. If you offered me the chance to go back to that caravan right now for a week, my bags would be packed within ten minutes. I have many lovely memories of my time with Sam there. For our wedding, I wrote Sam a poem called 'The Day We Met'. I have written a couple of poems and I'm fond of this and one other, which appears at the end of this memoir.

The Day We Met

The day we met,

I pledged my life, that one day soon you'd be my wife. That day is near, my life complete.

As man and wife our lips will meet,

then on a honeymoon we will go,

and leave behind the pomp and show,

a quiet week for just you and me.

We will sit and read just by the sea;

we'll make memories so fond and dear,

and laugh away our darkest fear.

Then will come the time to pack,

and onward home we'll travel back,

to the life that was meant for you and I,

happy forever until we die.

One evening, Sam's brother, Jay, came down from upstairs and was talking about online games. He played a game called *Unreal Tournament* at a competitive level. He told me about a new game being released called *Star Wars Galaxies*. It was called an MMORPG, which stands for 'massively multiplayer online role-playing game.' As he was telling me how the game worked in actual time with thousands of other players, I became enthralled. As soon as they released the game, I bought it and was hooked on online gaming. Sam played a little for fun but never got into SWG. After some time, the game died out and the now-famous *World of*

Warcraft emerged. Sam's brother and I played together for a long time, and finally, Jay played with different friends, so Sam and I started our own guild on our own. Before long, we had 120 active players from all over the globe in 'The Breed'. We all shared the same passion for games and would raid and hold fun events whilst chatting on comms.

Over the years, we have played so many online games and they have been an escape for us both; plus, we have met some lovely online friends. Later down the line, I played a game called *Eve Online*, which is set in space and you have to learn skills in actual time and make and fly spaceships. The game was hard-core and taken seriously by the player base. The story that got me hooked featured in a PC magazine about a disgruntled corporation (guild) being backstabbed by a group of other players. The head of the corporation wanted revenge and searched out a group of in-game mercenaries called 'The Black Hand Gang'. He paid them a vast amount of in-game money to destroy his enemies. It took the gang a year of orchestrated moves to become friendly with the group of enemy players and to be trusted by them to join them. The group became incredibly powerful in-game and after a year, their plan came to fruition and, when least expected, they struck. They killed the leader, who thought they were all friends. They stole every single piece of equipment, ships, assets, and in-game money, known as ISK. The plan had taken a year to execute, and it had gone spectacularly. They were told why they had done it, and the rest is the stuff of legends. The in-game value of the assets was £17K in real-world money, had they sold them, but it was not the money the group was after; it was the deception and meticulous underhand planning and revenge that motivated them. This was when I started playing *Eve Online*. As a newbie player, I was soon in trouble, and another player came to my aid and we began playing together. Every game I ever played from that moment onwards was always played with Steve. Sam and I got to meet Steve and his wife years later in Wales at the caravan. Over time, Steve and I became good friends and were there for each other during hard times.

I was becoming a bit bored and sat at home constantly, so I looked around for something to do as a hobby and stumbled across a Wing Chun club in Croydon. I went along for a taster lesson and decided I quite liked it. I liked that I became a bit fitter and was in time able to learn how to defend myself. Wing Chun is a form of kung fu and what Bruce Lee was first taught. The owner of the club was a bit of an arse, but I enjoyed the classes and progressed well, and after some time, I passed my fifth grade. Some drama ensued, and the instructors left, as did I. A couple of the instructors started on their own and I followed with them. The classes were more advanced, as they did not hold back any of the secret techniques . During my first grading, they awarded me a first or second, and my ego took a dive and I never went back. I was silly, really. I cut my nose off to spite my face. But I look back fondly on those times and on a couple of guys I trained with. It also gave me a little more confidence if ever I felt threatened.

We didn't have loads of friends in Wallington; I was close to Sam's brother, Jay, whom I would invite down to our flat every time we got a takeaway and we would chat about games for hours. I saw Hazel now and then, and we became good friends with our hairdresser, Jen. She was a sweet, affectionate, fun-loving girl, and after she left the salon to go into mobile hairdressing we became good friends.

Although I had taken no drugs for a while, Hazel was a huge pot smoker, and it was not long before I asked her to get me some. Jay was besotted with Hazel but not interested in the pot and frowned on us taking it. But the more Hazel popped over, the more he fell in love with her. Eventually, they got together, and the inevitable happened; he also began smoking pot. I regret that a lot, but I'm unsure how I could have stopped it. I wasn't into it but smoked it more than I should have at maybe three times a week. My mental health did not seem too bad, although in hindsight, it didn't help.

During this time, Facebook had arrived on the scene and everyone was busy adding old friends and acquaintances. One day I looked up Hailey's younger sister, Mandy. I sent her a message asking her how she was, and how my kids were doing. She told me that Hailey was struggling with them both and that they were a handful. Mandy thought it would be a great idea if I began seeing them again and I agreed and told her that was why I had looked for her. She told me she would suggest to Hailey to look for me on Facebook and suggest I could see them and maybe help with them. Hailey found me on Facebook, as planned, and we met at Danson Park in Bexleyheath in Kent one afternoon.

Chapter Twenty-Seven
My Children

That summer afternoon in 2008, we packed a picnic and drove to Danson Park in Kent, and at 1:00 p.m. we met Hailey, Mandy, my two children – Daniel and Josh – and their little sister, Maddy, from another father. I had not seen them for so many years. Josh was five, Daniel was eight, and Maddy, two. It was a shock to see them, and Hailey was even pleasant, which made life much easier. Mandy had three children of her own, all with their mother's fiery red hair. Daniel and I took Maddy for a push on the swings, and he told me I was fantastic with kids. It touched me. He seemed so mature for an eight- year-old, and he remembered everything from five years ago. Josh was a typical five-year-old boy, running around the playground, and he wasn't that chatty. I could see he did not know what to call me, as when Hailey referred to me as Dad, he shied away, embarrassed. Hailey told me they were both a handful, she was struggling with their destructive behaviour, and that they never listened to her. She told me that Daniel had ADHD, which meant he had boundless energy, and Josh had Asperger's, which meant he was not as sociable as other kids and preferred his own company. They were both lovely kids, and I felt a sense of belonging seeing them. The piece of me that had died five years previously grew back. We saw them again once every two or three weeks, and Hailey and Mandy hoped I could help with some stability in their life – that having their father back in their life might do them good.

For my fortieth birthday in 2009, all of our friends and family clubbed together, and Sam and I booked a week all-inclusive in Corfu, Greece, during the early part of May. This was our first proper holiday together for many years, and we were excited. The first few days were glorious and we soon turned red, and as the week went on, the temperature rose as well. We met some lovely people during our stay at Aquis Sandy Beach. The all-inclusive food and drinks were amazing, as was the entertainment team, who were all English. After the shows, a group of us, including the team, would sit outside and drink, and it was so much fun. On my actual fortieth birthday, I fancied a dirty pizza, so they arranged a takeaway to the hotel, and at 11:00 p.m. I sat on the porch of the bar, munching down on delicious pizza whilst getting drunk.

We became friendly with a couple who were in their early seventies. They had a profound sense of humour, so we chatted throughout the day whilst drinking coffee. One day, they told us about how the neighbours in the next room had been going at it the night before and that the bed had been banging against the wall. We all laughed, but it was only three days later when going back to our room and we met them that we realised they were next door, and it was us who were their neighbours. Sam and I died of embarrassment.

After one sunny day by the pool, when we went back to shower and put after-sun on, I noticed something odd. Sam had a very large handprint on her back. I put my hand up next to it, and it was much bigger than mine. It was a mystery where it had come from, as nobody had touched her that afternoon. We later referred to this as the hand of God. The hand was huge.

When we returned from Corfu, I began to feel I was becoming fat and lazy, so I started looking into different fitness classes, doing yoga once a week in Sutton with an experienced teacher named Milli. Milli was from Slovenia and tall, slim, and attractive. She was well travelled, and she knew a lot of Sanskrit from her travels in India and time spent with yogi masters. I went to yoga every week for over a year and became somewhat fitter, if not slimmer. I was going to the advanced classes after a few months and would sweat buckets during class. At the end of each class, we would lie down for fifteen minutes whilst Milli relaxed us into a slumber and would wake up feeling refreshed.

One evening, they invited me to a meditation evening in an old mansion in Guildford and it ran on so late. I had dropped Sam off with my mum and was late picking her up. On the way home in the car, she asked me, 'Are you fucking Milli?'

'No,' I said.

I was not, and after that, it became awkward. I stopped going to yoga. Sam wasn't a jealous person, so I took it seriously.

One day in the summer of 2011, Sam's brother, Jay, came downstairs. We had an argument, and sadly, it became physical; the police were called, and the shit hit the fan. Sam's family turned against us and I felt frightened living in my home. We signed up to home swap, and within six months we found a tiny bungalow in Cobham, but it fell through. We began looking again, and I was growing increasingly desperate, as I was scared living below Jay. My mental health took a really bad turn and I became quite ill with the stress and fear. If there is one thing I hate, it is confrontation or the fear of it. Once I get into a scrap, I'm fine. But the mental pressure of the anticipation of a scrap was getting to me, and I started to become a recluse. Every time I was out, I was worried about bumping into him and the repercussions. Eventually, we matched with a small flat in Coulsdon on an old mental asylum called Netherne Hospital in Netherne-on-the-Hill, which seemed ironically apt.

Chapter Twenty-Eight
Netherne-on-the-Hill

The flat was tiny and in a block of six with communal gardens and halls. The area itself was idyllic, with views over the Surrey Hills out of our lounge. The estate was part private and part social housing. It was a new build and architecturally was lovely to look at. Once we agreed to swap came the horrible task of packing, and we hired a man with a van fairly cheaply. The lounge was tiny and just enough room for our sofas, Sam's wheelchair, my desk, and not much else. The floor comprised a cold grey plastic industrial-looking tile. I stuck down laminate like sticky tiles and my dad was so impressed, he paid for it, which was lovely, and it made a vast difference. The kids loved us living in Netherne, as there were so many kids of all ages knocking about, and the times they stayed, they went out and kicked a football around on the field by our lounge. They made a lot of little friends in Netherne, and they had a lovely time running around in the fresh air every time they visited.

We had a need for a council occupational therapist, and we told her I was beginning to struggle with Sam's caring needs and looking after the home, so she set up a carers assessment with social services. I was becoming burnt out and everything was a huge burden for me. I got no day off. If Sam had diarrhoea in the middle of the night, she came first and I was just exhausted.

On top of this, my mental health was still a problem, with me hearing things and having anxiety. Social services visited and gave us an assessment, and they offered us twenty hours of help with agency carers. We gladly accepted, and soon enough, they came over four afternoons a week, assisting with some cleaning and helping Sam, which was much appreciated. A year after using the agency, one lady left and we took her on ourselves, paying her directly. Lilly was my age and from Mexico. She lived locally with her family and would come in and blitz our flat clean; she kept all our ironing up to date and was a marvel. At the time, we had a Motability car, and I would put Sam in the passenger's seat and fold her chair up and pop it in the boot. We had some nice cars over the years, with my favourite being the Nissan Qashqai. Banstead and Reigate social services were so good to Sam and me. Every year, they allocated us a grant for a holiday for us both, which was a joint respite. And we had some lovely holidays which we would never have had otherwise. I always felt so much more recharged when we got back, and we never took this for granted.

Before we'd moved to Netherne, our friend Jen was never far away and she would pop in once a week for a cuppa if she had a spare hour. Jen was one of my best friends and meant the world to me. Sam and I were going through a hard patch. We weren't making love and our relationship was becoming strained. I felt a lack of love, alone, forgotten, and that I was just Sam's carer, not her husband. It had all become about Sam's care and needs, and not about us as husband and wife. One day, I told Jen I had feelings for her. Jen was shocked and told me I obviously had problems in my marriage. Within a week, I realised Jen was right; I had an issue with my marriage and did not have feelings for her. I was lonely. I talked to her and apologised, and I promised I would tell Sam about this sometime soon. Jen had been single a fair while. I am not sure why – she was lovely looking and had an amazing personality. She was one of these single girls you look at and think, why are you single? She had a few drunken flings until one day, she went on a date with her personal trainer, Dennis. They were soon a couple, and he moved in with her. She rented a beautiful flat in Wallington and had been saving for years for her own place. We met Dennis once or twice, but I did not take to him. He was young, muscly, and wore designer clothes, fancy watches, and drove a Range Rover. Maybe I was just jealous, but I just didn't like him. I always wanted Jen to meet someone and be happy. The longer she stayed with Dennis, the less we saw of her until, when we moved, she didn't even come to say goodbye. I called her the day before the move, and she told me she was busy and to call her tomorrow. That was the last time I spoke to her.

Our time with the kids wasn't an easy one. The drive from Coulsdon to Bexleyheath in Kent meant using the dreaded M25, and you could never tell if the motorway was blocked full of traffic. I picked them up on Friday afternoons at school and dropped them back home on Sunday afternoons. The kids argued a lot; their bedrooms at home were pigsties. I would keep at them about making more of an effort, but they ignored me. Hailey would go in there and find countless plates and dishes under their beds. It was gross.

Hailey had a static caravan in Allhallows Park in Kent on a Haven site. She spent most weekends down there, so often I would pick the kids up from there. Maddy, Hailey's other child, was a sweet, shy little girl who adored her dad, John. John and Hailey had been best friends for a long time, but one night, she seduced him and then got pregnant. They tried to work things out as a couple many times, but eventually, he realised what she was like and moved on with his life. When I first met him, I was told he played *Star Wars Galaxies*, so I had a lot in common with him. I tried hard to get on with him, but he did not want to know me. During their times of turmoil, I tried to warn him, but he just couldn't see it, and she did to him what she did to me. Sorry, John, I tried with you. Last I heard, he had a nice place and a baby with a nice girl, so happy ending for him, I guess.

Our neighbours in Netherne were a mixed bunch. My ground floor neighbour told me he was an electrician and part of a notorious gang family. Allegedly, he had shot his sister's partner and had spent eight years inside. We had a few people come and go, and there were a couple of occasions where they would stumble in at two a.m. drunk and yelling, which was horrible. The funniest moment was when one girl, Stacy, who was around thirty-five years old, knocked at my door drunk as a skunk and told me she loved me. I told her I loved her back, and she staggered off . . . I wish I had given her an enormous hug for that; she was so sweet.

During our time in Netherne, we had two strange occurrences. During Election Day, I went up to vote in the local hall only to be told I had already voted. Apparently, someone had come in posing as me and gave my details and stole my vote. To say I was furious was an understatement. I could not understand why anyone would do such a thing, or what they would gain. The voting clerk reported it to the Electoral Commission, and the police were told, but nothing more could be done. Two years later, I spoke to the clerk before voting day. Luckily, she lived in Netherne. We arranged for me to come in first thing to vote, so if the guy came in, he could not take it, and the clerk would try to get CCTV footage of him. I went in first thing in the morning. I was told later that he did, in fact, come in and when asked if he had the paperwork, he said it was in his car and he walked out. As soon as he came in, the clerk called the CCTV operator and they got him on film. The police were called, but a couple of months down the line, nothing had happened, so I spoke to the lady, and secretly, she sent me a screenshot of him and a lady who had been with him. Finally, I could find out who had been impersonating me. As I looked at the picture, I realised it was my former neighbour, the electrician, and his aunty who was now living next door. I was shocked and could not work out the motive. I told the lady who they were, and the police came round and they took a statement. I was asked if I wanted to press charges and stand up in court, but not being well at the time mentally, I didn't feel strong enough to do that. I was happy for him to be cautioned, though. He never explained his crimes, but in all honesty, I think he just wanted to fuck with my head a bit. The funniest part was when speaking to the policewoman, I told her about him saying he had murdered someone, and she told me that if he had done something like that, he would not get a warning. The only time someone would get a warning was if their record was clean. This meant he had not murdered anyone. When I realised this, I laughed to myself at how sad someone must be to impress people with that kind of sad shit.

We had not long moved into Coulsdon when Sam began suffering from terrible spasms in her legs. The pain was so awful that I had to call an ambulance. They admitted her to our local hospital in Redhill, Surrey, and as luck would have it, her consultant came and saw her in the ward. He told Sam he was applying for an alternative medicine called Sativex, which was medicinal cannabis in spray form. It had to go to a panel to be signed off and was a difficult drug to get prescribed. It controlled Sam's spasms well, but she got some horrible symptoms. She was so dosed up, she was a bit of a zombie, and one day, she told me she had heard voices. I was proud of her to have the courage to tell me, and we stopped it. It took a few months, but her health improved with no symptoms and she never took it again.

In autumn 2012, Sam got an awful chest infection and was confined to bed. It was so bad that our GP and district nurses called in palliative care from a nearby hospice. We were given a hospital bed which we put in the lounge, and Sam was in so much pain that they put her on a morphine pump. We were also calling the district nurses out twice a day for them to give her booster morphine injections for extra pain relief. Things came to a head during the summer holiday. We had the kids over, and I had called our doctor out. She took me outside into our communal hallway. 'Darren,' she told me, 'You need to prepare yourself; Sam will not make it to the end of the week.' I was told the same thing by one of the specialist hospice nurses, too. I was so angry and confused – how could Sam be dying? She was chatting to me. The thought of being left alone in the world without Sam seemed worse than death for me. I would not cope alone – what would I do? I suffered silently. I felt like a fraud telling my family the news, as I did not believe it. That afternoon, I sent the kids out to play and sat down next to Sam and told her what they had said to me. She was furious at our GP for telling me that. She called the specialist nurses and told them in no uncertain terms to get the morphine pump off her and that she was having no more booster injections. Sam would later tell our lovely lady GP off about what she had told me and that it had worried me, and I chuckled. That is the spirit, I thought. Sam knows how to fight. She was so slim and frail, and her eyes were slightly sunken in. But she had made her mind up that she was going to recover, and she did. She made a full recovery. Our niece, Lilly, was born slightly after and Sam was well enough to visit my sister and have a lovely cuddle and a picture taken. It was a wonderful moment for us.

One Sunday evening in late 2013 when I was driving the kids home, they were chatting together and told us that there was something they wanted to tell us. A couple of years ago, there had been an incident at their caravan where Daniel and Josh had gotten into a fight. Josh had picked up a knife and attacked Daniel and, in the process, had stabbed Daniel's foot. Afterwards, Josh had hidden under the bed, and they had rushed Daniel to the hospital. A police search went on until they found Josh. At the time, I had been very disappointed in Josh's behaviour and had told him so. But what the kids told us next shocked us. They told us it was Hailey who had attacked Daniel with a knife, and afterwards, in a panic, told them that Josh must pretend it was him, otherwise social services would take them away. I did not know what to think, so I asked them if they wanted to tell the police and said they could stay at ours for a bit. They said they did, and so we drove to a police station, and statements were made. The police visited Hailey, and I took them back home to Sam and my place. A CID detective investigated the case, and because they'd already involved social services with Hailey, they took out an order, meaning she could not see them for their own protection. The kids' Aunty Gail agreed to have them both until it was all sorted out, and between us, we muddled through. After a few meetings with social services and the police, and charges were dropped. The detective believed Hailey, and they dropped the case. The kids still maintain to this day it was their mother. Hailey could have them back, but there was so much tension in the house afterwards, and every time I called or picked them up, all you could hear was screaming and swearing. It was a shit atmosphere for the kids to grow up in.

At this point, Daniel had passed his 12+ and was given a prestigious place in the county's best grammar school, Beth's. But he could not handle the discipline and was too immature to understand that destructive behaviour would not be tolerated, as he was disrupting the class. Eventually, he was expelled, and his mum got him a place in a tiny special school run by a mum for her kids. But Daniel's behaviour was still bad, although I believe he was happier at Safe School. Eventually, he was asked to leave and ended up in a delinquent school in Thamesmead. It was a vile place where dropouts ended up, but he had a couple of decent teachers who mentored him, and over a year, he integrated back into mainstream school, albeit one day a week. He was soon back into school, put back a year, but seemed to settle in. Josh was still in little school but preparing to enter senior school, and my frayed nerves calmed down.

My mental health had been wonky for a little while, and in 2014, I was seen by the Croydon CMHT (Community Mental Health Team). After what seemed to be an eternity of waiting, we finally saw a registrar psychiatrist. He wanted to take me off all meds and see all of my symptoms. With all the meds I was taking, nobody knew where I was or what my original symptoms were. I was put on aripiprazole (Abilify), which was a new antipsychotic. It did not agree with me at all, and when we went up to Wales to visit Sam's parents, I began having awful social phobia and panic attacks just being around people.

One afternoon, I drove my father-in-law down to the shops in Carmarthen and was so shaken up, I had to ask him to drive. We sat in the car park at Home Bargains and I shook like a leaf with anxiety and fear. I was popping herbal antianxiety meds called Quiet Life, but I was not having a quiet life . . . I was going through a terrible life.

We got back home, and I was determined to not let it stop me from going out. I was trying to quit smoking and would pop down to the local vape shop for supplies and could not pick the vape juice up from the counter, my hands shook so badly. It made me feel like a freak, and I was petrified by everything. My gut told me to stay in and not go outside, but I felt I should fight my anxiety. I begged my GP to take me off the Abilify, but he wouldn't and told me it had to come from a consultant. I asked for appointments with him, only to be told there were no consultants to see me. They trapped me on that med for a year and a half.

That time was a living hell for me. My voices were still there, and I was paranoid that Sam was cheating on me. It was during this time that I asked Sam to come clean to me and I would with her, as I felt wracked with pain and paranoia. She told me she had never cheated, and I told her I never had either. I did, however, tell her I thought I'd had feelings for Jan for a week, and that hurt her. Had I been well, I would have mentioned nothing, but I was poorly and felt compelled to reveal this to her.

We changed carers a few times, although we stayed friends with them. One girl we employed in 2015, Sophia, was a vivacious girl who was fun to be around. I was getting into photography and had bought a Canon DSLR, and I showed her how to take some nice shots of flowers. There were two issues with Sophia: one, she made me manic to be around; and two, she was a terrible cleaner. One day whilst in the throes of mania, I wrapped Sellotape around my head so it distorted my face. We found it hilarious, but Sam did not and struggled to cope when I became like this. We visited one of my consultants shortly after, a lovely older gentleman. Sam told him she was worried about my mania and so he asked her for an example. Sam brought up the Sellotape incident, and he chuckled. I asked him if he would like to see the picture I took and he obliged. Two minutes in, the consultant and I were still in fits of laughter, much to the dismay of Sam, who told him, 'You both need locking up.'

We took Sophia on holiday to Egypt, as I found looking after Sam and the travelling exhausting, but it didn't work well. Sophia treated it as a holiday for her, not as work, and I fed Sam rather than us taking it in turns. Sophia got drunk a few times, which was fine, but one night, she was plastered and puked all over the bedroom floor. I had to stand her over the toilet whilst she upchucked, then put her to bed. I then spent the next hour and a half picking up pieces of pasta that she had vomited under our beds. Hotel rooms rarely come with a mop, so I had to improvise with towels, and it was horrible. She woke the next day, oblivious to the night before, and it was only when I showed her the pictures that she realised how she'd behaved. The day we turned up at the hotel, I felt unwell, and my voices went into overdrive for no reason I could think of. I stopped eating for three days and felt quite distressed. Every time I got in the shower, the voices were screaming for me to fuck

Sophia. I kneeled in the shower praying to God and all the saints to save me from what seemed like demons hell-bent on destroying my life and those around me. I tried as best as I could to enjoy myself, but it was difficult. One lunchtime, an attractive girl came over to our table and said, 'Hey, Darren, how are you?', then walked off. Here we go again, I thought, weirdy-weird stuff happening. Who was that girl? How did she know me? Every time we went to eat, I would look out for her. After four or five days, we saw her again and she told us she was the travel agent we had booked with, and I recognised her. She looked different in a swimsuit and no glasses.

I have happy memories of the shishya bar, sitting in a mock-up Bedouin tent, and riding a terribly tempered camel called Sue. There was one annoying server in the complex who latched onto Sam and would not let go. We saw him a few times, and he would come over to us and serenade her. The first couple of times, I told him we were married and to leave us alone. It was creepy and in poor taste doing that to a married woman in front of her husband. One evening, as we were walking out of the restaurant, he came up and began his singing to her, and it was like flicking a light switch. I yelled at him she was married and to leave her the fuck alone. I then went and complained, and for the next two hours, all we could hear was him and the hotel's general manager yelling at each other. I think they sacked him, although I hope he wasn't and that they just told them to wind his neck in. Shortly after getting home, we told Sophia that we were letting her go; she wasn't up to the cleaning, and with my voices and mania, it was not fair on me. We felt awful, as Sophia was a nice girl and she had a lovely son whom we had met many times. We employed another lady soon after and funny enough, her name was Sophia too. She seemed bonkers, too. It was the name.

One of Sam's dearest wishes was to move back to her home in Wales. Although we had fun there, I never wanted to move there. It was grey, it rained a lot, and was full of Welsh people. But we agreed to put our names down on the council list with a very strict set of criteria. We asked for a two-bedroom bungalow with a garden in a small town with shops and somewhere to grab coffee. It took about two years, but in late 2016, we received a phone call from one of the specialist housing teams in Wales telling us a bungalow that might suit us had come up. We asked Sam's parents to go view it to see if it was worth our coming up to view it.

They gave it the thumbs-up, telling us it was in a friendly and quiet town called Llandovery in Carmarthenshire in South Wales, known for its sheep festival. So, we planned for Sam, my mum, and me to stay with Sam's parents and view it.

Chapter Twenty-Nine
Wales

When we arrived at the bungalow, the weather was grey and dull. We met the housing officer, builder, and occupational therapist and went in for a look. As I pushed Sam around, we realised it was lovely and had a lot of potential. The OT measured the doors and told the builder about what adaptations we would need. The bungalow had two bedrooms and there was a large double door between the two bedrooms so I could push Sam into the spare room. In the spare room were patio doors out to the patio back garden. The back garden was small, but large enough for us to put up a shed, flowerbeds, a barbeque, and a table to sit outside. The lounge was quite small and because the door into it was small, I struggled to get Sam in. The occupational therapist asked the builder to knock down part of the hall wall, which would open the lounge up with no door. The bathroom was a tiny wet room but would suffice. The kitchen was a decent size with room for appliances, and that led into an outhouse and out to the garden. Sam could not get out this way, which is why they had added the patio doors to the spare room. We stepped outside, and I asked Sam if she liked it. She told me she did.

My mum agreed we would never get better, and not in Surrey, where we lived. I had to agree, the bungalow was perfect. The town had a small co-op supermarket, lots of pubs, and many other shops and cafes. It ticked every box on my move list, so we decided there and then to take it. The housing officer told us it would take about six weeks to finish the work. There were bits we needed to do ourselves, such as the floor. It had a concrete floor throughout except for the kitchen, which had a tired vinyl floor. We decided it would need a laminated floor for Sam's wheelchair. A carpet would not last five minutes. We priced up a nice oak laminate and I got a quote from the carpenter working on the place to fit it. The floor cost us £1,250, and it cost £650 to fit it. It seemed silly to pay so much for a nice floor and then for me to do a shit job laying it, and with furniture down, it would have been a nightmare. We took out a credit card and paid for the floor, and once again, my dad came to the rescue and offered to pay the carpenter to fit it. He did not need to pay for that. It was a kind gesture.

We packed up our little flat in Netherne-on-the-Hill and told those around us we were moving to Wales. The news upset a few people, including our current carer, who would lose her job, and our friend Jen, who was upset. She told us she could not travel up to see us with her work. I felt sorry for our carer, but what could I say? We had been on the council list for two years. The day arrived to move, and we were mob-handed with all of my family turning up on my doorstep.

The date was 24 September 2016. My sister and brother-in-law hired a massive lorry with a tail lift, which they swore was much bigger than we needed, but it only just fit everything in, including three cats in travel boxes. The drive to Wales would take five hours, but my poor brother-in-law Richard called us to say the lorry had a speed limiter fitted to it and it would only go up to fifty miles per hour.

We all arrived in Wales and began unpacking. It had been a long day, and we were exhausted, but it did not take us as long as I thought it would to get the basics done. Things like books and keepsakes could stay boxed for now. By 6:00 p.m., we had had enough, and so my mum went out and got us a takeaway. We knew that there was an Indian restaurant, two Chinese takeaways, a fish and chip shop, and a kebab/burger place. I went out with my mum. It was cold, dark, and raining quite hard, but our little town was heaving with people out for the night. Every pub we walked past had awnings out and music or bands playing. There were people out and about everywhere, drinking and singing. We picked up our food and when we got back, my mum told everyone how busy Llandovery was and what a lovely sociable busy town it was with bands out in the pubs. We soon realised that we had travelled down during one of the largest events in Carmarthenshire that weekend, the Llandovery Sheep Festival. Revellers from far and wide would visit the town and there would be stalls up, pubs filled to the brim with people up for the weekend to celebrate an old Welsh event. We laugh about it now – how lucky we were to have bands in our little town for our arrival.

The carpenter had laid our floor, and with all the extra work the council had done, our new home looked amazing.

It took some time for social services to set up a new carers package, but we were soon employing a lady to come in three times a week. She only lasted six months, though, and began using odd excuses to not come in, so eventually, we let her go. We advertised for another carer and were fortunate to find a lovely lady named Marion. She was older than me and lived in town with her son. She had four children, and they had grown up and moved away. Marion was a breath of fresh air. She kept our place clean, doing all our laundry, and she also spent a lot of time taking Sam out. Once a week, they would drive out to one of the larger towns like Brecon for an afternoon of shopping, followed by tea and cake in a nice coffee shop. Over the three years Marion was with us, we became good friends. She had a lot of friends in town and introduced Sam to more and more people when they went out for walks, sometimes ending up in a cosy pub for a cheeky vino.

My health had not been good for a fair while, and in 2018, I was diagnosed with type 2 diabetes. It meant more tablets for me, but I took so many as it was, I did not even think about these new ones. My family came up regularly to visit for a few days, staying in local pubs for the weekend. I soon found that if all of my family came up together, I struggled to cope with them all, and the visits felt chaotic and exhausting. So, after a few visits, I asked them to come up as smaller groups, like just my mum and one sister.

My children were soon growing up. Daniel, my eldest, started university in 2019, studying PE. In the first six months, he partied hard and worried the living daylights out of me, but then he met a lovely girlfriend, and calmed down. He managed to find work in a local pub and began saving for a car. My youngest son, Josh, had started college to study to be an electrician. He enjoyed the college course and told me he found the work easy. He was extremely fortunate that a friend of the family knew a guy with an electrical engineering company, and a call was made, and Josh began volunteering with them. Josh worked for this company twice a week for free for a year, just to gain experience. I was so immensely proud of him. After his first year of college, they took him on as an apprentice and paid for his college.

Since moving to Wales, my depression declined. I visited my GP, who suggested I see the local CMHT, but they would not take me on their books, as I was told I was not ill enough. I felt that my mental health was being ignored by the consultant, so I just went back to my GP, who changed my antidepressants from 60 mg fluoxetine to 30 mg duloxetine. I began getting problems with pain in my testicles. I was treated occasionally for epididymitis, which is an infection of the testicular tubes and quite painful. For a long time, Sam and I had problems with our sex life. Sam could not feel it due to nerve damage and had no libido. I had no libido and suffered from erectile dysfunction, using blue pills to help. We checked my bloods for my prolactin levels, which can cause a drop in men's testosterone, and yes, my antipsychotic was causing high levels. They gave me testosterone gel to rub into my skin. In May 2019, my mental health had deteriorated and Sam insisted on visiting my GP with me. The GP told me that my testosterone levels were still low, and my Testogel was not working, so I stopped using it. I was kind of glad, as my testicles had shrunk a lot and I still had no libido. Sam insisted I see the consultant, because she felt I was poorly and not coping. I was very depressed and had no motivation; I was constantly fatigued and did not like leaving our home.

Soon, we had an appointment with a lovely lady psychiatrist who listened to everything Sam and I had to say. She promised to make an appointment with the CMHT and told us we would be seen by a CPN as well. Sam was very clear that I needed a support network.

The day the appointment came in 2019, we had to visit another surgeon, and as I sat in the large waiting room, I could not face being around or seeing other people. I felt anxious, so I put my head down and covered my eyes. We were called and shown into a small room, but seven professionals sat in there. I could not cope with the large group, so I told them and four of them shuffled out, leaving Sam and me with the consultant, a female CPN, and the lady psychiatrist from before. I told them how I had been feeling, and the consultant began asking me if I had felt sluggish, depressed, etc. I informed him that I felt I was struggling with life and had become so withdrawn, I did not want to live anymore, even if I had no plans to kill myself. I felt wretched, but I could not bring myself to leave Sam on her own in the world and have to go into a home.

The consultant decided on a med change and was quite open with me about what our options were. He asked me if I'd like to try a different antipsychotic drug called quetiapine instead of my Amisulpride. I was asked if I had tried it before and I told him I didn't think I had and was prepared to try it. They wanted to start me on 50 mg and go up every week until I reached 400 mg, so it would take me two months to get up to dose.

My new CPN, a nice girl called Kit, spoke to me once a week to see how the med change was going. Honestly, it was going badly. I spent a few weeks tapering off Amisulpride, and then on Monday, I started 50 mg of quetiapine at 8:00 p.m. with the rest of my meds. By 10:00 p.m., I could barely stand, let alone lift Sam out of her wheelchair and onto her commode and then onto the bed. As I went to lift Sam, I lurched left and right as if I were drunk but somehow transferred her. I spent the next few days lying on the sofa. I wasn't sleeping but just lay there with my eyes shut, waiting for time to pass. It was a horrible experience, and I felt like I was slowly dying. I was so exhausted, and every muscle and bone in my body throbbed and ached. I did not eat throughout the day, but at 10:00 p.m., I became ravenous and ate a shocking diet of crisps and chocolate. By Saturday I felt better, and then Sunday I was back to being fine again. I was horrified at how the week had gone but was told side effects would subside, so I increased it to 100 mg the next Monday. I felt no better and spent two months on the sofa, save Saturdays and Sundays where I felt somewhat more human. I hoped I would get up to the therapeutic dose and would get used to the effects and be okay.

June and July came and went, and our home was a disaster area. As soon as Marion tidied up and cleaned, I would make a mess and not be able to clean up after myself, so the poor lady was firefighting. This made me feel awful, knowing I was causing problems for her and not being able to do anything about it. During this period, I also felt sick, too. My testicles hurt, and I went back to a few GP, who told me it was chronic prostatitis, and I was given hard-core antibiotics for two weeks at a time. I was also referred to the chest clinic, as I had been coughing and getting very out of breath. The chest clinic appointment was over a four-month period and comprised various tests and scans. After all the tests, the respiratory consultant told me I had mild emphysema and needed to give up smoking. He told me that the cessation smoking clinic at the hospital had an excellent success rate and that he would refer me. Here we go again, I thought. During my MRI scan, they found an incidental fatty benign tumour 5 cm by 4 cm by 3 cm in the back of my shoulder. I was told I would have it scanned every six months to make sure there were no changes, and it was harmless.

I was also having a strange panic-attack-type thing going on. If I became stressed, I shook and my breathing increased, but my heartrate did not change at all, which baffled my GP. He could not see it was a panic attack without the racing heart, though, as I felt very anxious every time it happened and out of breath, too. It happened during a GP appointment and he took my oxygen levels and said they were fine and to monitor it. Also, I was having many odd symptoms, such as my tongue going black down the sides. It was quite sore, but nobody seemed to know what it was and they just told me to monitor it. I was also becoming thirsty in the evenings and up all night peeing, so I popped back to the doctors, who asked me to take a blood test. My blood sugar levels gone from 52 to 108 within a few months. So they gave me more diabetic medications, and I was told to watch what I ate, which didn't help, as I was too exhausted to cook and was only eating crisps and chocolate unless Marion cooked me a decent homemade meal, bless her.

I was back and forth to my doctors every week because of my prostatitis, in so much pain I could barely sit, and I was getting frustrated and cross. I asked one of my main doctors what I should do about it and he told me to get on with it and if I was in pain, he would give me more antibiotics. I went home and the next day took advice elsewhere. I found a website that helps men with issues with cancer in their reproductive areas. I spoke to a lovely specialist nurse who, when I told him what was happening and how the GP had told me to get on with it, was horrified. He told me I needed to ask to be referred to a urologist as a matter of urgency. I began feeling that I was just an awkward patient, but also frustrated and like I was being fobbed off. I spoke to another GP, and he referred me to urology. I asked him if what had happened with his colleague should upset me. He said little and muttered. They offered me a testicular scan to check for tumours and I was thankful that it came back all clear.

After two months on the sofa, I got to the max dose, and it seemed obvious I would not tolerate being on quetiapine. I had a visit from my CPN to tell me she was handing me over to a colleague because of work commitments. They gave me a new CPN named Rod. At the time, I was trying to smoke tobacco, as I could not afford normal cigarettes. My sister Jennine used to work in Belgium a lot and would bring hundreds of fags back for me, and I would pay her for them. She hadn't gone for a long time, and I found a guy on Facebook who sold fakes and tobacco. I regularly bought some; now and then they would be vile, and I would sell them on Facebook for the price I'd bought them for. There were lots of people in our town selling duty-frees and fakes and I tried a few, but I could not get on with baccy. I bought some baccy to sell locally from the Facebook guy and sold some, but it became dry and people stopped buying it, which meant I had a few leftover. I had also been so desperate for cigarettes myself, I had found some dodgy Polish bloke on a Facebook selling site selling Polish fags. Sam and I drove to the Llanelli, and I bought £400 of cigarettes. When we got back and I began smoking them, I realised they were vile and could not smoke them. I felt so stupid, as Sam had warned me not to buy them, but I didn't listen. Like the tobacco junkie I was, I needed my nicotine fix. I tried to sell them on all the Facebook groups I could but could not shift them, and Facebook began clamping down on the sale of tobacco, as selling duty-free or fakes is illegal in the UK. They consider it a soft crime, though, as it doesn't hurt anyone, and when times are hard, you do what you can to scrape by. Smokers have had money gouged from them by the government for years with tobacco duty. I smoked a very cheap brand and they cost me £8.65 a pack, and I smoked two packs a day. About £6.50 of that is tax, which is extortionate to charge an addict who will pay whatever it costs to get their legal fix of the addictive tobacco. It was an easy tax on those of us who could not stop smoking and were an easy target. I had some baccy leftovers and gave some to Kit, who smoked. I told her I had the Polish fags if she knew anyone that wanted to buy them, and she told me Rod might.

Rod seemed pleasant enough, too, but Sam and I had taken to Kit. She was so bubbly and helpful, and she seemed like she really cared. I spoke to Rod about coming off the quetiapine and trying something else. It was decided that I get back down to zero for two weeks and then taper onto something else like risperidone. I had tried risperidone once many, many years ago and had only taken it for one night, as it made me feel fluey the next day to the point I could not get out of bed, so this idea did not please me much. They decided that I would spend two months tapering down at 50 mg a time. I developed a lot of problems with my stomach and was told it was IBS; I had diarrhoea and tummy aches for a few months, and during this entire episode, I pulled my shoulder and had to have a steroid injection into the joint. I felt very sorry for myself, as I was physically and mentally broken.

During my time coming off meds, I felt Rod was not supportive of me and didn't care. He didn't return my calls, so I called up the team one day and asked to change CPNs and go back to the girl. I was told a meeting would be held the next week and they would bring it up. A couple of weeks later when I called, the receptionist told me that my CPN had not changed and I still had Rod. I felt bloody stupid and awkward; I'd made a complaint, and now I was stuck with him. I left it for three weeks but eventually manned up and called him. I explained it wasn't personal; I just felt like Kit had cared more and I felt like he didn't and was not even returning my calls. In all fairness, he agreed to carry on and said he would meet up with me to see how I was progressing. After the two months tapering off, I felt so much better mentally, as my brain fog had cleared and my energy levels had increased. When speaking to a lovely old friend with schizophrenia, I told her I had been med-free for a week and felt great. She told me to think about staying med-free and I balked in horror. I had not been med-free for twenty-three years, and the thought horrified me. But I felt great and had heard no voices for a long time. I spoke to Rod, who told me he would speak to my consultant but agreed I should try it. I asked for my new med to be on standby at brief notice if things took a downward turn.

After three weeks of being antipsychotic free, I felt great with no symptoms of paranoia, no delusions, and no voices . . . just beautiful silence. A month turned into two months and then into three. I believed I may be okay and that a miracle had occurred and that this was a second chance . . . a miracle from God. I told Sam I had every intention of grabbing the opportunity with both hands, and I was going to do whoever or whatever had made me well proud and not fuck it up.

Chapter Thirty
Christmas 2019

Life seemed on the up. I had been off meds a while and my mood was buoyant. We spoke to my family in late October about our coming down to Surrey for Christmas and seeing everyone. We would stay at my mum's and she said she would sleep on her sofa. Everyone got excited, including me. At the start of December, our eldest cat, Shadow, lost lots of weight and was skin and bone, so we took him to the vet, where they did lots of tests and found out he had an overactive thyroid which was speeding up his metabolism like crazy. We were told he would have felt pretty awful, and we put him onto meds which I had to give him twice a day. At the same time, we had all of our large bills in and I panicked about our money. We sat down and worked our finances out.

With the new large vet's bill for £180, we decided we needed to cancel our Christmas visit to my family. I spoke to my mum first, who was obviously upset but understood. I called my sister Jennine, and she had a real go at me about cancelling. I was not in the mood for anyone to chastise me for cancelling because of something I had no control over, so I had a go back and put the phone down. I could not remember falling out with either of my sisters to the point of not talking to them. It quite upset me that she didn't realise I had no choice. I called my mum, who told me she was just disappointed we weren't visiting, but as I told her, my sister had never lived close to the edge financially, so she would not understand what it was like to live on government benefits and that this £180 broke us.

I noticed some changes in myself: I was getting my old mojo back. My energy returned slowly, I didn't feel as anxious going out, and doing chores at home wasn't as difficult. Sam and I spoke about triggers that might make me unwell again, remembering a situation where I was in a supermarket and two older women had walked past me and one had turned to the other and said, 'Darren isn't well at the moment and we are worried.' She could have been talking about her son or grandson. This would be an obvious trigger for me, and we tried hard to think of a way of being ready for it. We decided I would just have to talk to Sam if it happened again. In the three months I had been off antipsychotics, I had not heard voices and could not believe what a miracle it was. I felt like I had won the lottery, but better.

We got up on Christmas Day and I gave Sam her present, a nice bottle of Adore perfume. She had seen the advert on TV and told me it was her favourite, so I'd saved up and bought it. I also bought her a Bluetooth headset with a mic so she could chat on comms with our online gaming friends. We had said to each other that we would not buy each other gifts at Christmas, but when she gave me a bar of chocolate, I was upset. I know I shouldn't have been, but I felt it was thoughtless not to get me anything, regardless. I had dropped some hints about having a back massage over December and had bought our carer Marion a £50 voucher with our local massage lady. My mum called, and she was with my sisters with all the family and I spoke to everyone, including Jennine. I got off the phone and told Sam I was going into the bedroom. I lay on the bed next to Lulabelle, one of our cats, and cuddled up to her and wept.

Whenever I felt like shit, I would go to Lulabelle and she would always welcome me with furry kisses, and I knew she loved me no matter what.

On Boxing Day, because I was in such a shit mood, I put Sam in a shit mood. We took down our tree and every decoration. That was it.

Our Christmas was over, and I turned my back on it.

Chapter Thirty-One
The Year from Hell

On 3 January 2020, I had my PIP benefit face-to-face meeting at home. I was a nervous wreck when the lady sat down; I put my hand over my face to cover my eyes as I told her the things she wanted to know. I thought it went better than my previous interview. She seemed thorough and was at ours for a long time. But I later found out they only offered me a standard living rate and nothing else. It meant we were £100 short a month. I had taken a PIP online test a charity had provided, to give you an idea of what I should get, and it had told me higher rates on both living and mobility. I was disappointed to put in for a mandatory reconsideration but knew it would be months until I heard anything back.

The week of 6 January 2020, one evening it was late and I was smoking in my kitchen, as I always did, checking my mobile for any notifications I might have when something unusual appeared on my screen. My screen time had flashed up, and when I noticed a website about asexuality, I balked, wondering what it was. Within a couple of minutes, my paranoia was peaking as I saw many sites on my phone I had not visited. Some sites frightened the life out of me. There were a lot of links for login sites for the government, the County Council, and Trading

Standards Wales which had been logged into every day for the three weeks, going back before Christmas. I was like a dog with a bone now. The deeper I delved, the more I was sucked into a rabbit hole of paranoia and psychosis. I told Sam, and she didn't seem concerned. We went to bed, and for the first time in a very long time, we made love. Sam felt pleasure, and the intensity reminded me of years gone by. I could not believe we actually made love . . . normally.

The next day, I spent time researching all the sites that had come up on my phone and decided to screenshot everything in case I needed evidence at any point. I spoke to my friends from *World of Warcraft* on comms and told them about what had happened, and my first thought was that it was the DWP (Department for Work and Pensions) putting me under surveillance for the face-to-face assessment. My friends laughed at me and told me not to be silly and that I had just been hacked. That night, Sam confronted me about why I had been so quiet all day and looking up things on the web. I had told her about it the night before, and only now she was concerned? We had a blazing row, and she screamed and shouted at me that she was going to have me locked up and that she should have called the police because I was losing my mind. It hurt to hear Sam say these things to me, and using the hospital as a solution to what was going on pissed me off. She told me if I didn't stop, I would ruin everything. But I had been sent mad many years ago by the 'police' at Paradise Club. It would not happen a second time – like hell, and this time I had proof of foul play.

That night I could not sleep, and my mind was running ten to the dozen. I got up and wondered why Sam was being horrible to me. Did she know something I did not? I sat down at my computer and looked at her Facebook site via my account. I went through all of her posts and friends, trying to find anything that shouldn't have been there. My mind was playing tricks on me. Was she having an affair? Was she in on something?

The morning came, and I was exhausted and a mess. I contacted Apple support, and they guided me to their senior team, who began looking into what had happened. I was told to change the password on my Apple ID, which I did. They seemed to think somebody had access to my account and so we added in F2A authentication, too. Cheerful things had been fixed, I turned in for the night, hoping the next day would be happier, but when I got up, I saw that the activity on my phone was continuing. It looked as though the access was at midday, 6:00 p.m., and midnight. If this had been some young hacker mucking around, I could not see him logging on for three weeks at set times; they would have been at random sporadic times, and therefore, I did not believe it. I called Apple back, who were surprised, and they asked me a lot more questions, and eventually, they advised me to reset my password again. At this point, I was a real mess. My voices had returned, and I was paranoid as hell, too anxious to go out.

Covid-19 hit, and the government began talking about lockdowns, not going out, and self-isolating. We were due a new Motability wheelchair car, a beautiful Peugeot Rifter. We were lucky that they delivered it a day before lockdown, although we had to follow social distancing rules. It was at least one piece of good news.

On 23 January, I went back to my GP. My feet were very painful with a burning, tingling, numb pain. He looked at them and told me it was because of my diabetes and gave me some pregabalin meds to take. I got home, and we had Sam's OT and physio over to see her. I told them what was happening, and they said it could be the meds and not my mental health. The next day, I started the gabapentin, and after the first one, I got very confused and by mistake took five instead of three and became poorly. The morning after I took one, I realised it was my meds making me confused. A week later, I called my CMHT and spoke to Kit. I was so panicked on the phone, and she told me I could take some

Valium if needed. She told me that some meds have what is called a paradoxical effect on people doing the opposite of what they're prescribed to do. I was very anxious and panicky, and it took me about ten days to get myself right. Over time, the GP increased my duloxetine to 120 mg to help with my nerve pain.

My mobile phone was still showing strange activity, and I called Apple again. The support worker asked me to upload the screenshots for him to check out. He sent me a link to my email, but every time I clicked on the link, I had an error message: 'Site Forbidden'. He was as confused as I was and asked me to send all of my data from my account for one of their teams to look at. I got off the phone, terrified, and later decided to call him again, so I went to the Apple support logo on their website. Every time I clicked the 'Call Me' button, I had the same error message – 'Site Forbidden'. I genuinely believed whoever was behind this had hacked my computer system, too.

Another scary thing was that two sites that had been recorded had been removed from my phone over the whole three weeks, and that was the Council and Trading Standards Wales. I had taken screenshots, or the proof on my mobile would have gone with that. The only person who had any of our details was Rod from when he had visited and had had no signal. He had asked me for my Wi-Fi password. I didn't feel comfortable giving him access, but he was a professional, so I did. You can bet that I soon changed my router and Wi-Fi password. I reformatted my computer and deleted my Apple account and had my iPhone just as a mobile. While sorting all of this, I had an issue, so I called up support and explained everything that had happened. They asked me for all of my reference numbers and told me they had no record of my incidents, even though I had the Apple emails in front of me. . . . Gee, thanks, that didn't freak me out much, either.

Screenshots below.

..ıll Club 📶   22:04   24% 🔋

❮ D M's iPhone   **Other**

~~Daily Average~~   ~~10m~~

Updated today at 22:04

APPS & WEBSITES

	Amazon	❯
	eBay Shopping – Buy and Sell	❯
	argos.co.uk	15m ❯
	asexuality.org	15m ❯
	carmarthenshire.gov.wales	15m ❯
	currys.co.uk	15m ❯
	my.dchs.nhs.uk	15m ❯
	peacocks.co.uk	15m ❯
	retail.santander.co.uk	15m ❯
	thefragranceshop.co.uk	15m ❯
	tradingstandardswales.org.uk	15m ❯
	theweatheroutlook.com	5s ❯

LIMITS

.ıll Club 🛜　　　22:06　　　24% 🔋

‹ Screen Time　　**D M's iPhone**

‹　　Wednesday, 08 January　　›

- 　30m
- everydayhealth.com
  30m
- google.co.uk
  30m
- icy-veins.com
  30m
- mayoclinic.org
  30m
- my.dchs.nhs.uk
  30m
- peacocks.co.uk
  30m
- retail.santander.co.uk
  30m
- store.steampowered.com
  30m
- thefragranceshop.co.uk
  30m
- tradingstandardswales.org.uk
  30m
- FaceTime
  25m

..ıl Club 🛜	22:07	23% 🔋

‹ Screen Time   **D M's iPhone**

‹   Saturday, 04 January   ›

- 🧭 retail.santander.co.uk
  — 6m ›
- 🧭 store.steampowered.com
  — 6m ›
- 🧭 thefragranceshop.co.uk
  — 6m ›
- 🧭 tradingstandardswales.org.uk
  — 6m ›
- 💬 Messages
  — 5m ›
- 💬 Messenger
  — 3m ›
- 📧 Outlook
  — 3m ›
- 🧭 certforums.com
  — 3m ›
- 🪙 Coinbase
  — 42s ›
- ☁️ Weather
  — 19s ›
- 🔍 Indeed Job Search
  — 14s ›

.ıll Club 🛜 22:07 23% 🔋

❮ Screen Time   **D M's iPhone**

❮   Friday, 03 January   ❯

- tradingstandardswales.org.uk
  26m
- FaceTime
  17m
- Clock
  5m
- betterhealth.vic.gov.au
  3m
- WebMD: Symptoms, Doctors, & Rx
  2m
- rightsnet.org.uk
  2m
- gov.uk
  2m
- healthline.com
  2m
- whatdotheyknow.com
  48s
- Coinbase
  37s
- Outlook
  17s

| Club 📶 🛜   22:08   23% 🔋

‹ Screen Time   **D M's iPhone**

‹   Friday, 03 January   ›

- store.steampowered.com
  26m
- thefragranceshop.co.uk
  26m
- tradingstandardswales.org.uk
  26m
- FaceTime
  17m
- Clock
  5m
- betterhealth.vic.gov.au
  3m
- WebMD: Symptoms, Doctors, & Rx
  2m
- rightsnet.org.uk
  2m
- gov.uk
  2m
- healthline.com
  2m
- whatdotheyknow.com
  48s

.ıll Club 🛜   20:26   33% 🔋

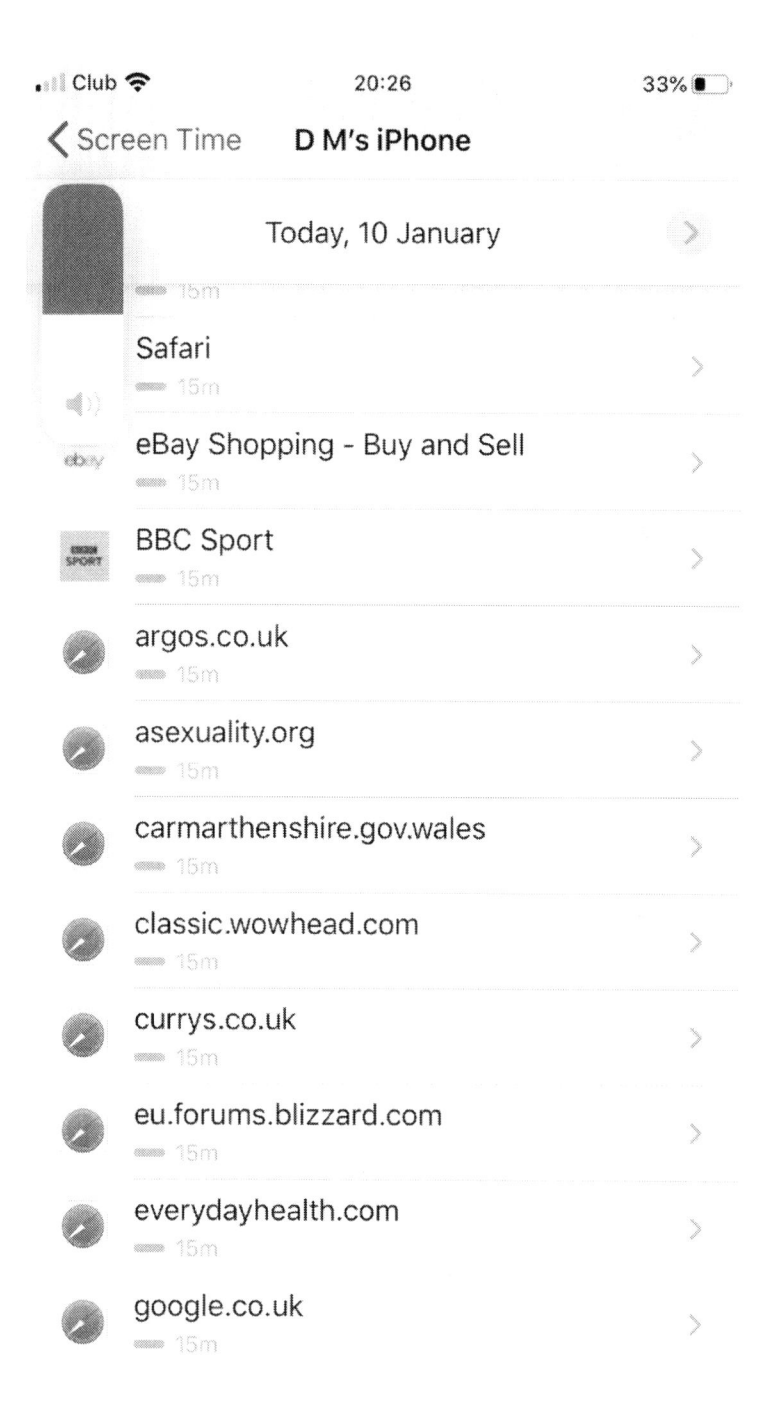

‹ Screen Time   **D M's iPhone**

Today, 10 January   ›

Safari — 15m   ›

eBay Shopping - Buy and Sell — 15m   ›

BBC Sport — 15m   ›

argos.co.uk — 15m   ›

asexuality.org — 15m   ›

carmarthenshire.gov.wales — 15m   ›

classic.wowhead.com — 15m   ›

currys.co.uk — 15m   ›

eu.forums.blizzard.com — 15m   ›

everydayhealth.com — 15m   ›

google.co.uk — 15m   ›

Chapter Thirty-Two
The Voices

During the crazy few weeks at the beginning of 2020 after this breach, my voices came back with a crash. In fact, it all came back, although I beat the paranoia off. A few weeks later, and I decided that this would not beat me. I vowed I would fight tooth and nail for my sanity. I began writing positive notes in my diary that I could go back to. I was terrified, upset, paranoid, anxious, and I found hearing voices painful – it was like mental torture to me. I decided I would not be afraid of going out or worry about being under surveillance. If I was, screw them. Every time I went out, I was petrified to the point where I shook, but I kept my chin up high, and if anyone looked at me, I smiled at them. I also slowed down my pace and began looking around anywhere I went rather than rush around with my head down. I made eye contact and smiled. After doing this for a month, my paranoia went.

My dominant voice was Annabelle with many other minor voices, both male and female. I had heard Annabelle the first time twenty-three years ago but thought she had long gone. She screamed at me, and in my mind, I screamed back. I was living in two different realities: one on the outside with Sam and actual life, and one on the inside with them, and it was exhausting. I was working hard to keep our place cleaner, looking after Sam, and trying to fix all my mental health problems, or, as I would say to Sam, 'I'm in the office with the kids.' They spoke in themes, and the themes changed every few days. As the theme changed, so did the voices. The themes pertained to the police, the hospital, a CPN, the Pope, ex-girlfriends, angels, high society, demons, God, time travellers, sexy aliens, telepaths, the secret service, and the axis of evil. They had an amazing imagination. To begin with, it seemed like they judged me for about three weeks. Every day, my past actions were mentioned, and I felt like I was atoning for my crimes. I asked God for forgiveness and I learnt to forgive myself; I asked those I had wronged to forgive me, too. I had to explain all of my crimes and transgressions to the voices, and eventually, it ended. I did the same for my voices and I forgave them of their sins towards me. I pictured Annabelle as I closed my eyes. She was a dark sooty demon sitting in a large cave with a small opening of light on the top. As I spoke to her, I began forgiving her and the things she had said to me that had hurt. I also rubbed her body in the cave with a metaphorical cloth. After fifteen minutes, I stood back and could see that she was a giant metallic-blue dragon with golden wings and claws. She was beautiful, and I told her she could be anything she wanted in life. This was a fresh start. So, flying up to the opening in the roof and feeling the sunlight on her wings, she gently flew off. For two days, Annabelle was like a sweet teenager, kind and pleasant. The other voices still talked, but my main one seemed happy.

I had called to God for help many times. I asked for an angel one afternoon and an unfamiliar voice came through to me, but with a metallic note to it. She told me she was an angel of the Lord and not to worry, no harm would come to me. I asked her name, and she replied that I could call her whatever I chose. I named her Aziraphale after an angel from a book I had once read. We only spoke twice, but she reassured me that God had a plan for me and not to worry. One of the other voices said, 'He has a countenance with God', and I did not know what countenance meant, so I had to google it. When I read the meaning and context, it quite surprised me that a voice had used a word that was unknown to me, and that its context was correct.

Within less than a week, Annabelle went dark again and told me it was her choice. She spewed vitriol at me, calling me anything she could. She wished a painful death on Sam, and I was so livid that I cursed her. I vowed I would be there when she died and I would look her in the eyes as she gasped her last breath and she would see me. Thinking back now, I was in a horrible place, and now the thought I could curse like that is quite dark. But if pushed past the breaking point, even a placid man will erupt.

I started thinking spiritually about what I was going through and Sam told me that many years ago when she was young, her mother had taken her to a spiritual church called the Chapel of Light, where she'd had faith healing. After the event, she had gone home and had red handprints over her body even though they hadn't touched her. We looked up the church and found their website. It wasn't far, so we checked the timetable and they were open every day for faith healing. We set the date, and the following Monday we set off. The weather was horrendous with torrential rain and wind, and as we drove on, the car was low on petrol, but close to the town we found a petrol station, so we grabbed a sandwich and a drink. When we got to the church, there was no parking, so I got out of the car and went to check the gates to see if I could park inside the church car park. I walked up to the gate and realised they had shut it. I checked the front door – locked. I was confused and annoyed and needed the toilet. I walked around the back, and the place was shut up. I walked around to the front again, and on the board it said it should be open. There was no note on the door, so I tried the mobile numbers, but no answer. I was angry with them. We had driven an hour in terrible weather for nothing. When we got back, I left them a message on Facebook, and it was seen later but they never got back to me, so I called them again and left a message. It took them a week to get back to us and they spoke to Marion, our carer, and apologised, telling us we could go down any time. I was so angry, thinking they could shove their hands-on healing.

Annabelle began tempting me, and she offered me various roles in life. Would I like to be Jesus, an angel, would I like to win the lottery, did I want to be an undercover police officer, a secret service agent . . . I just had to choose and accept. I declined everything and told her they would not buy me and they would not tempt me. In my mind, had I accepted winning the lottery, it would have been like compensation for what had happened to me and selling out, and I was not accepting that. She spent three days telling me about a highly classified programme founded by Pope John Paul II, Princess Diana, Nelson Mandela, and George W. Bush. I was told that a small group of people had been chosen to be given telepathy and would be trained to work for an agency for the good of humanity. I still declined, even though I believed they had created it for good. I told her I did not believe voices were natural and wanted nothing to do with them. You may ask why I would believe such a thing. But when you hear a voice speaking to you like an actual person would, it is impossible to not believe it. What amazed me was the fact that Annabelle spent three days building up to the offer and, using my powerful sense of morals, tried to snare me by telling me respectable people had formed the agency, such as Nelson Mandela. I had the occasional friendly voice. When I asked for help, a female voice told me to go outside and get some fresh air, and for her I was grateful.

In late January, my voice went very hoarse and croaky. I had an earache and a pain in my jaw, so I went to my GP, who told me it was laryngitis, and it would go within two weeks. About six weeks passed and I was still in pain, so I went back for a second opinion from a different doctor. I was told it was just laryngitis and that it would go on its own.

With this and my chronic prostatitis, I was in a bad way and had lost faith in my doctors but did as I was told and went away. After twelve weeks, I was at the end of my tether, fed up with being fobbed off by my doctors, and went and saw a third doctor who sent me for a blood test to check my thyroid. It came back fine, so he told me he was sending me for an emergency appointment with an ENT. Because the Covid lockdown had just started, he told me that I would not be seen for a very long time, and I felt let down. The next day, however, I received a call from an ENT consultant asking me about my symptoms. I explained that my throat was sore, my voice hoarse, and that I had ear and jaw pain. He made an appointment for me to go down to outpatients within a week, where I would see one of his registrars. The lockdown meant that the hospital was like a ghost town and everyone was masked up. I had a camera put up my nose and down my throat, the registrar finished up, and I was told I had a lesion on my vocal cords and was shown a picture. I was quite worried and asked him if they could remove it. He told me it could be lasered off, but he would like to get me back within a week for a biopsy under a general anaesthetic. I was fortunate that they gave me a pre-op after my appointment with him, and they advised me I would hear within a few days about the operation. A few weeks passed, and I called the ENT department to be told that all operations had stopped until further notice but that I should be fine for twelve weeks. The GP who had sent me also reassured me I should be fine, too, and as soon as lockdown allowed, I would be fast-tracked. During this time, I joked with Sam that I was going to heal myself by holding my throat and visualise myself healing the lesion.

From February onwards, I realised I was not sleeping as soon as my head hit the pillow, so I cuddled up to Sam at night, and after making love, I felt a little closer to her. We began going to bed earlier and putting our salt lamp on and lighting a few scented candles with music. It was quite nice, and we became more romantic again, trying to be intimate more often. Sometimes it worked; sometimes it did not. We also downloaded a couple of meditation apps to help us chill before bed. I felt loved again.

After my non-event with the spiritual church, I emailed the Vatican and my local parish priest in Llandovery. It was a detailed email, and all I wanted was some spiritual comfort. Maybe a nice mail back from the Vatican, and I was hoping the priest would call me and pop in for a chat and a cup of tea to talk through my concerns. That did not happen, though. An hour after sending it to him on Facebook, I had a call from the Carmarthenshire Police saying a call had gone in for my safety and they wanted to know if I was going to harm myself. I was embarrassed and angry. What about a priest's confidentiality? My local priest called the cops on me. And my email was intelligent and coherent – see below. So, let's say my faith in the church has gone down the toilet of late.

Chapter Thirty-Three
My Email

To whom it may concern,

I have no idea where to start, so please forgive me. I need advice concerning things that I cannot explain happening in my life. I apologise for the long backstory, but I think it applies to what is happening to me at the moment.

I led a fairly normal childhood in the UK until the age of thirteen when my parents began a nasty violent divorce. I spent a long time in despair and hurt. At twenty-four, whilst I was studying at university, my long-term girlfriend left me for another man and broke my heart. I took the break badly and went off the rails. Sadly, I mixed with the wrong crowd and I turned to drink and drugs. It was not long afterwards I became psychotic and ended up in a psychiatric ward for five months, where I was treated very badly. For the last twenty-six years, I have been diagnosed with schizoaffective disorder and have been heavily medicated. Since the moment I became ill, I have tried to lead a clean moral life, not only because it was the right thing to do, but for a clean conscience.

For many years I could work, find love and a normal life. I cannot even explain some horrors I bore witness to, from voices, shadow people, synchronicity, delusions of grandeur, and awful paranoia. I realise that these are all common symptoms of my condition and were nothing more than terrible mental illness. I have accepted a responsibility that it was my choice to take drugs and then become unwell.

When I was thirty-three, I met my current wife, and it really was love at first sight. The moment I saw her, I knew within a split second I was in love with her and wanted to spend the rest of my life with her. She was in a wheelchair with a condition called Friedreich's ataxia and was reasonably well. Over time, my wife gradually deteriorated, and I gave up work and have now cared for her for fifteen years. I have made it my sole purpose in life to care for and love my wife. In turn, my wife has always tried to support me in my struggles with my condition.

Three years ago, we moved to Wales in the UK, and I asked my doctor to refer me to my local Mental Health Team. The psychiatrist I saw refused to take me on until three years later when I became unbearably unwell. Last June, they changed my antipsychotic medication to quetiapine and the side effects made me unwell, to the point I spent four months on the sofa unable to do anything. I decided to taper my medication off and was told I had to be off them for a couple of weeks before a new antipsychotic could be slowly added in. During the time I came off my medication, I felt well mentally, although my physical health went downhill very quickly. A friend with a similar condition told me to consider staying off meds for a short while and see how I go. I suggested this to my psychiatric nurse, and he agreed. It has been five months since I have been med free, and until four months ago, I had no mental health symptoms.

MY CPN has told me I have been misdiagnosed for twenty-six years and did not have schizoaffective disorder but, in fact, had drug-induced psychosis and that the enormous amount of medication was probably making me unwell. I did not need medication for much of the past twenty-six years. During the period of coming off meds and my mental health improving, I have become unwell physically: chronic painful prostatitis for nine months, IBS, my diabetes has gone through the roof, and I now have neuropathic pain in my feet. I ache all over my back, I am breathless, and have been diagnosed with emphysema. During a CT scan from the respiratory consultant, they have found what they think is a deep intramuscular benign tumour in my shoulder and laryngitis that will not go. I have to laugh about my health and have told my wife I am fully expecting leprosy next week.

My doctors have been quite poor in the treatment of these conditions and I have had to push quite hard to be referred. About six weeks ago, I noticed unusual behaviour on my mobile phone, and on inspection it became clear something was very wrong. There were sites that had been logged on my phone that frightened me to the core, like government sites, Nation Health staff login sites, a Parliament archive site . . . I could go on. (Please find attached for your curiosity.) It sent me into a panic, and for over a week I suffered from paranoia, anxiety, and a tremendous amount of stress. I reported it to the authorities and Apple, whose technical team was genuinely concerned. At one point I could not even access web pages on the Apple site . . . the page said 'Forbidden 403'. To say they were surprised is an understatement. Thankfully, I had screenshots of the sites on my phone, as two days later, some sites they visited disappeared off my mobile. I called the police, who were not in the least bit interested. I believed I was under surveillance . . . this triggered a traumatic week. It has taken me some time to get over the incident and my CPN has told me I was 'gaslighted' – by whom, I have no idea.

I am now symptom-free apart from one, and that is voices in my head. Hearing voices is an explainable symptom of serious mental illness. What I have found curious, however, is the fact I am not delusional, I am not paranoid, am not depressed, manic, and rarely get anxious. So here I am, perfectly fine, except I am hearing voices. I believe nothing the voices tell me, and I believe the only reason I can do this is because of being ill for twenty-six years and having gained insight and experience. I do not want to hear them and honestly want nothing more than to live a normal happy good life.

Please take everything below with a healthy pinch of salt, as I believe nothing that is said to me. They are a mix of friendly voices and evil voices. The friendly voices are kind and calm and have even given me tips on how to make them quiet. The evil voices try to tempt me with various 'offers,' such as winning the lottery, being Jesus, the secrets of the universe and even a job, using telepathy, with a secret agency. What astounded me about a voice in my head offering me a job was the sheer detail, and the meticulous intelligence that went behind it. The voice used my own strengths against me, my strong morals to do good, and for days would not take my no for an answer. The voice tried to make me think a group of good, moral people made it . . . of them was Pope John Philip II. This led me to believe the job was to do good. I still declined, as I feel voices are unnatural . . . even if it was true.

One voice came to me yesterday, and she declared she was an angel and here to guide me through my problems. I asked her name, and she told me I could call her whatever I liked. She told me that no harm would come to me and that she would guide me when needed. While she spoke to me, I felt a tremendous sense of relief and a sense of calmness and that all would be well. She also had a unique quality to her voice that I just cannot explain.

For my sanity, I believe that the voices are a part of my subconscious created because of severe stress. But it is abundantly clear that some are good and some are evil. If you believe that evil actually exists as any form or entity, or whether you believe that the devil is real and does actually tempt people, as he did Jesus in the desert, then I hope you will be open-minded and at least consider what I am going through to be something other than a single symptom of mental illness . . . maybe it is a symptom, but they differ from when I was psychotic. They are lucid, normal sounding, and I can hold a conversation with them easily.

If I am perfectly honest, I do not believe in much, apart from accepting God into my life, purely as a defence mechanism and to keep me grounded. I can tell you I am not delusional; I do not believe I am anyone other than an ordinary person going through things that I cannot make sense of. I do not want any attention; I just want to live a normal life. I really have no idea where to ask for help. I honestly have no idea how to move forward and could very much use your divine wisdom. Now I am unsure if I will get a reply, be told to speak to my local priest, told to see my CPN, or be taken seriously as someone of interest to the church . . . and somebody you can help.

As an afterthought, it is quite obvious to me that evil very much has a foothold in the world. It seems like people are asleep and nobody cares anymore.

I really hope you reply to me soon and may help me.

I hope his Holiness Pope Francis forgives me of any wrongdoing.

With much hope,

Darren Smith

Chapter Thirty-Four
Spring 2020

As I changed after going off meds and fighting my voices, I became more organised. I started writing post-it note lists every day to keep my mind organised and busy during the day. My personal hygiene improved, and I became more active around our home, keeping it much cleaner. I knew Marion was struggling with the demanding work involved, and just after Christmas, she told us she was thinking about looking around for an easier job. We understood completely. I told her I was trying to make more of an effort, and she told me she had noticed.

I was coughing and choking a lot because of the smoking and having emphysema, and it had stained my fingers dark brown. I was so ashamed of anyone seeing my fingers that in the shower I would use a pummel stone to get rid of the stains. My fingers would be quite raw, but I was so ashamed. I bought a glove to wear when I smoked so my stain would go. I went through four gloves in four weeks, as the heat went straight through the glove. Finally, I became so fed up, I called the smoking cessation team at Glangwili Hospital and was given some NRT patches and nasal spray. I read up as much about giving up smoking as I could and bought an herbal tincture called lobelia which binds to the nicotine receptor and helps stop cravings. I also bought a book from one of the country's leading advisors on giving up smoking, a guy named Professor Robert. In his book, he advised making a video for yourself to watch if ever you feel like having a cigarette. I made a video which was incredibly raw, and I hate watching it back. I was coughing, spluttering, and explaining why I hated smoking. I emailed Professor Robert, and he emailed me back and gave me some great encouragement. I sent him a link to my video, and it quite took him aback by how powerful it was.

On 24 March, I stopped smoking. I had explained to my smoking specialist that every time I had tried to quit in the past, it got harder the longer I went, until five or six weeks in, I was pulling my hair out and ready to cut my wrists. The craving pain I had in my chest was excruciating, and knowing that one cigarette would take it away was just too much and I would cave in. The first couple of days were odd. I sat outside with Sam, and we timed how long a craving lasted, and it was between ten and fifteen minutes. I drank a glass of water and waited it out, and it passed. The lobelia helped, as I realised when I cut it down later down the line. The days turned into a week, into a month, but I was still cautious about whether it would get harder as it had every time before, but it did not. After seven weeks, I realised it would not go the same way and felt relieved. The entire time I was quitting, family and friends congratulated me on my progress, but I shrugged it off in case I jinxed myself. I felt like I was running a marathon, so I did not look back at how far I had come, and I did not look forward . . . I kept my head down and just kept running.

A week or two later, I called Rod, my CPN, and he just answered with 'Yes?' and not 'Hey, Darren, how are you?' or 'How is the med change going?' It happened again a week later, and I was so incensed that I called the team, made a quiet complaint, and asked to speak to the office manager. He called me and I explained how I felt Rod did not care about my welfare and how he didn't return my calls. It was just unprofessional, and I had had enough. He told me he would change my CPN from Rod to another guy called Jed and would speak to his team about their attitude about caring. Their method of taking messages changed, and henceforth, the message would be sent via email to the person so nobody forgot.

By April, my voices were causing me so much distress and I could not cope. It was constant, and I was being sucked down various rabbit holes of delusions. I spoke to Jed, who asked me if I would like to try a tiny dose of my old med, Amisulpride. I had nothing to lose, so I agreed. I was prescribed 50 mg at night and took it for three nights. I was shocked at the difference it made to me. The side effects of a starter dose were horrendous. I woke up aching all over, felt fluey, foggy headed, and lethargic, and worst of all, I craved cigarettes badly. By day three, I was pulling my hair out craving cigarettes, and it had only been for the three days I had been taking it, so there was no doubt it was the antipsychotic. I spoke to my mum on the third day and she told me to get off it, as going back to smoking was not an option. I stopped taking the Amisulpride, and it took a week before the craving went back down to its normal levels. I was so appalled by this that I made some inquiries. I emailed Professor Robert, who told me there was no analysis into the effects of smoking addiction and the use of antipsychotics, and he did not seem to want to champion the notion. After speaking to my smoking specialist, she told me that a med like that should help me quit, not the other way around. I asked her, If a drug addict had his dopamine levels reduced a lot, how would he behave? 'Oh, he would go cold turkey', I was told.

'So, if you gave that drug addict an antipsychotic which reduces dopamine, he would go cold turkey?'

'Oh yes, he would', she told me.

I was quite cross about this, and nobody seemed to care. There was no research on the subject, so what could I do? I emailed the Department of Psychiatry at King's College London, which specialised in research into addiction with antipsychotics. I had a lovely research doctor call me for a very long phone call where I explained what had happened. She seemed intrigued and told me yet again that there was no research. I argued that many antipsychotic medications on the market warned that gambling was a known side effect of taking them, which would point to my theory that lowering dopamine by some antipsychotics caused or worsened addiction. She told me she would do some homework and get back to me. I emailed her a few months later, and she told me they would not pursue it. I should imagine that if Big Pharma had a medicine that makes quitting an addiction even harder, it would not be the common knowledge you would want on your med leaflet. I'd done my part and passed the information on, and I could do no more. The establishment did not care to care. I tried lowering my mood stabilisers, lamotrigine, but within five days I felt suicidal, so I just put it back up. At this point, I had been antipsychotic-free for seven months, but the voices were taking their toll on me, and my morale was taking a beating. Every morning when my alarm woke me up and I went to the toilet, the voices would start, and I began to despair.

My birthday came and went in May, and I was still struggling, so I spoke to Jed about trying an old med I had liked called Stela zine. I started on a tiny dose of 2 mg and worked my way up to 7 mg. I felt I had lost my battle with the voices; I had been off meds for four months, and now they had beaten me and I was back on meds. My PIP had come through and I had only been awarded the standard rate of living allowance, meaning I was £100 worse off each month. I had put a lot of work into my mandatory reconsideration, but when I received the decision many months later, they refused me any more money. I decided I would take the appeal to a tribunal, which would take six months.

At the end of May, I was offered an appointment at a local private hospital to ENT to take a biopsy of my vocal cords. When I had seen the consultant in February, I was told I had a growth but not to be too alarmed. He had booked me in for an op within two weeks, but with lockdown, all routine appointments had been cancelled. I was grateful when the restrictions were lifted and I could go. When I went, the consultant told me that the lesion had vanished as if it had never been there. I joked with him that I had healed myself. In hindsight, I am sure it was because I had given up smoking.

I had not eaten chocolate for a little while and I gorged on a few bars one day. The next day, my tongue was so sore and I wondered if it could be chocolate that was making my mouth hurt. After some experimenting by not touching it for a week and then eating some, I realised I had become intolerant to chocolate. I had finally figured out one of my mystery illnesses and was disappointed but pleased at the same time. I also realised some cakes with too much sugar had the same effect on my mouth. We had solved the mystery of my black tongue.

I increased my Stela zine to 15 mg, which is considered a therapeutic dose for schizophrenia, but I began to not feel quite right and my paranoia returned at night after I had taken it. Jed was cross with me for going above the agreed 7.5 mg, so I eventually dropped the dose and stopped it.

The voices continued, although it wasn't all bad. Whilst lying in bed, I had a few very serious conversations with various unique entities. Some of my voices told me what they were. One night, I spoke to demons who wanted answers to some riddles. Who came first, the chicken or the egg? 'They came at the same time', I told them. Also, why did the chicken cross the road? 'Because he could' was my answer. I cannot remember the other two questions, but they liked my answers and told me they would never bother me again.

Another night, I chatted to a couple of female voices for a few hours and was told they were from our future and now lived in our time. They were open with me and we had a normal conversation. They told me they were housed in a bunker in a small port in Herzegovina. I had since googled it and found that there is only one port in Herzegovina called Neum, as Bosnia is landlocked. Neum is having millions poured into the town toward infrastructure, but no secret underground bunkers show on Google Maps. I was told that in the future, they had forgotten how to be human, so they had come back to learn. They told me they were much taller than us, but I cannot remember much else. It was an interesting chat that lasted a couple of hours. We then said our goodbyes, and I never spoke to them again.

On another occasion, I spent about four hours talking to a girl called Christine who had entered the British Secret Service and was using telepathy to communicate secretly. She told me she had signed up for the service and further down the line was handpicked for her role. She told me that part of her training included controlled chemical psychosis for six months, and it was quite horrendous. I spoke to her supervisor, who called herself Alias Sue, and she said she would like me to sign up, as I was a natural who had most of the training already. The only problem was that they wanted me to go to an address of their choosing to sign up. I declined and told them that, as a sign of good faith, I wanted a letter or note posted through my door I had to reply to. It could be anything, just as a sign that they were for real. I was not turning up to a random address in London and telling them they had called me in, no way. The next day came and no paperwork or slip came through, so I guess it was more bullshit.

The year went slowly with lockdown in place. We were all too frightened to go out, even up to the local co-op. Marion, our carer, stopped coming to work for six weeks, worried she may catch Covid and pass it on to Sam. She did slowly come back but kept her distance, bless her.

During the summer, I felt less and less appreciated by Sam and more like an employed carer. I spoke to Marion about it one day and Sam caught on that something was wrong and wanted to know what. Marion spoke to her, and we had lots of tears. I told Sam that I felt unloved by her, with no affection or kisses or hugs. Six weeks passed and things boiled over again. The lockdown had taken its toll on everyone – nobody was going out, and Sam was stuck indoors, too worried to go out in case she caught Covid. One day I had just had enough and spoke to my family about how Sam was cold towards me, how she had not changed since our last chat, and how I felt lonely and unloved. I'd been up all night fretting about us, and in the morning, I decided it was best if we split. I called up social services and asked them to find somewhere for Sam to move out to. They were kind and told us they would find somewhere the following day for her and offered me accommodation for the night elsewhere.

Sam sobbed her heart out all day and called Marion, who spent the afternoon packing her clothes. It was the most awful thing I had been through since being with Sam. At 6:00 p.m., Marion left, and I sat down in the lounge with Sam and we began talking. We were both heartbroken, and I realised I couldn't live without her. We hugged and cried into each other's arms all evening. I could never live without my Sam. The next day, her dad came over and talked to us, and I aired my grievances. She never kissed me or caressed me anymore, yet when I walked past her, I would pat her shoulder or kiss her head, and all I wanted was the same in return. Ron explained to her it was the little things that kept a marriage going, and we decided that now and then Sam could call me over and just ask me for my cheek to kiss. It made all the difference to me.

Even five months later, Sam was still hurt by our rocky patch and the fact that I'd asked her to leave. I have told her it wasn't something I wanted, but that I felt I was at the end of my tether and just needed love and some appreciation. I am sorry to have broken her heart, but I had suffered for years with these feelings and they had to be put right. My love for Sam had never wavered, but I felt very under-appreciated. Since caring for Sam, I have learned compassion and service to others is an honour. I am proud of how I feel I am giving something back to life, rather than taking anything.

My prostatitis was causing me so much pain, and I was back and forth to the doctors' still. They gave me the same two- week antibiotic treatment, and that evening I could not sleep. The next day I got the same facial rash as before. I looked up the side effects and not only found that a facial rash was common, but so was insomnia and hallucinations. I stopped the medication and wondered if it had contributed to my symptoms. The longer I stayed off it, the better my mental health got.

Chapter Thirty-Five
The Voice of God

In April 2020, I was struggling with depression, and the voices were making me have suicidal thoughts. One evening, I was sitting at my computer desk with Sam behind me on her laptop. I called out to God in my mind, as I had done frequently, and begged God to come to me. The next thing, I heard the loudest voice boom in my mind: 'I will be with you when I am ready.' I was quite taken aback and shocked at how loud it was, but I said nothing and sat there for ten minutes before deciding I needed the toilet. I sat down on the toilet, and it happened again. No mistaking the booming voice of God. I trembled, not in fear, but in awe of his presence. I told Him, 'God, I am trembling.'

And He said to me, 'The humble always tremble.' An evil voice started, and God told me it was coming from the bathroom light and to turn it off. I did as I was told, and the voice stopped. 'I want you to teach,' God told me. 'And I want you to write your book.' I told him I would do as He asked. He then said, 'Welcome to the family of hope', and left. I have not spoken to Him since.

It is so difficult to describe the experience. He had no accent and His voice sounded calm but commanding, not old yet not young. But when

He came, it was as if the volume was at the max, and I cannot explain how I felt in His presence . . . I was just in awe, and I trembled and shook.

After He left, I walked into our lounge and sat on the sofa arm close to Sam. She asked me what was up and I could not speak. My mouth was wide open as I sat shaking for twenty-five minutes. After I could speak, I told her what had happened, and I sat there, stunned, in clinical shock. It took two hours to wear off and shook me up.

From that moment onwards, I would push to get this book written. I thought I might have become more religious after what happened, but I didn't. But I felt immense frustration at what was happening in the world with Covid and felt I had been singled out by God. I thought it was my duty to do something. I did not feel special at all – quite the opposite. I was sure I was just a man going through a battle between good and evil and I was caught up in the middle. Sam and I speak about that evening now and then, and whilst she doesn't believe me, she is unsure about what happened. What is in no doubt with her is how I was afterwards, not being able to speak and being in shock for two hours, feeling numb and tingly. I guess thinking about it, I feel very humbled that He visited me, and welcoming me into His family was amazing.

About a month later, I was praying for a cure to Covid and a voice appeared to me and told me to help find a cure. I had to buy two amulets of hope and put them together. Nothing more was said, so I began looking for amulets. I told Sam, who made me laugh and told me to stop wasting our precious money on foolish items. I joked with her that as crazy as it sounded, if it cost me a few quid to do the bidding of a voice to cure Covid, I would, even if it sounded silly. I have two favourite saints in my life – the first is Saint Francis, and the second is Saint Jude, one of the forgotten apostles, often confused with the apostle Judas. Saint Jude is the patron saint of lost causes and the impossible and is said to bring hope to wearers of his amulet. I had found what I needed and bought two amulets from the Catholic store online with some holy water. I keep one on my mantelpiece with the holy water and my small thirty-year-old Bible. The other one is in a small pouch with a prayer in my phone with my cards and ID, always close by. I have a lot of admiration for both saints and how they conducted their lives. Both were holy men. I did not bring an end to Covid, but I felt better for doing as I was told, as it was a good cause.

In May 2020, I tried my Stela zine again and worked back up to 7.5 mg. I felt well enough to play video games, although I still felt poorly with an earache, a lack of energy, and was achy and a bit depressed. I did, however, begin upcycling our bedroom furniture, and we got a local guy in to decorate. So, I was achieving something tangible. I had an MRI scan on my shoulder and was told that my benign tumour had not grown and that I would be seen again in February. This was quite a relief. By September, my prostatitis was so bad that I went back to the doctors and saw a different GP. He offered me the same two-week antibiotic I had been given before and I asked him about the rash on my face and the side effects from meds, including psychosis. He told me they were not side effects and gave me the prescription. When I got home and read the leaflet, it mentioned a rash, hallucinations, and insomnia, and it made me quite cross with him. I highlighted the side effects on the med leaflet and when my CPN Jed visited, I showed it to him. He said little, but I do not think it impressed him. I binned them.

In September, I was told about an online counselling service in America called BetterHelp. You answer a questionnaire about the issues you have and what you would like from a counsellor and it then matches you with one. I had wanted to try therapy for a long time, but in the UK, prices are about £70 a session and way beyond my reach. I signed up and was paired with a kind lady named Melissa. She listened to my story and offered me valuable advice. After the first month, I told her I was struggling to afford the payments. She advised me to email BetterHelp, which I did. They came back with a huge discount, because I was not working. It meant I could get counselling for £23 a session, and I was very grateful for it. I told Melissa about my parents' divorce and how traumatic it was for me; I then explained the bullying, and how alone and upset I felt in life. It was a relief to get things off my chest, and after eight weeks, I felt as though I had come to the end of my sessions. I was asked to write a review, which I was more than happy to do, and a few days later, because they were pleased with my review, they offered me 'swag' and I chose a free T-shirt . . . nice touch, BetterHelp.

Come October 2020, we began looking for two new carers and we had three ladies apply. I interviewed them and we offered two of them the job. One lady started but she only lasted three hours. She told us she felt ill and went home, only to text us the next day that she was not suited for the job. We interviewed more people and had a lovely lady named Erin start work, and another waiting for her DBS security check before starting. It was so nice to have company in and to take Sam out again once a week. She also helped me keep our home clean, which gave me a bit of a break.

By November, I had really felt well for the first time in a long time. Mentally, I was not hearing voices much, and I felt optimistic about how things were going. Our second lady started shortly afterwards, and we got on well with both. Both girls were bubbly, hardworking, and good company.

Christmas of 2020 was a quiet one for everyone, as we were all put under strict lockdown. We still had a lovely day. I set the table for us both and cooked an enormous meal with chicken and ham. Sam had bought me a Samsung Galaxy 3 smartwatch, and I had bought her some diamond and sapphire hoop earrings in white gold. The UK looked forward to seeing the end of 2020, hopeful for a better new year. With 2021 came the rollout of two new vaccines. It was a light at the end of the tunnel for us, and the public became more optimistic.

Two weeks into January, I decided to try lowering my Stela zine antipsychotic. I went from 7.5 mg and am currently down to 2.5 mg, which is miniscule. I felt slightly stronger in my mind, so I also decided to try to quit smoking. It is a fight I am willing to have to be addiction-free. My forever dream is to be antipsychotic free with no symptoms. Time will tell, and if I have to increase my small dose of meds again, then I will.

In January 2021, I did have a strange occurrence. I was sitting next to Sam on the bed, and I told her I was trying hard to be the person she needed, i.e., more patient and less frustrated, when a voice came to me and said, 'He's incongruent.' I had never heard of the word in my life, let alone had a clue what it meant. I sat down at my computer and googled its meaning. It has a few meanings, but one that captured me was that when someone is trying to be the person they want to be against the person they actually perceive themselves to be, it causes conflict, anxiety, and pain. This is known as incongruence. I felt a little spooked by this but sat there and chuckled to myself when the same voice came back and said sarcastically, 'And this is why he is family.'

Part of me is optimistic about my future being off meds and having no side effects like voices, but part of me wants the voice of God to come back, as I have questions for Him this time. What does God want me to teach? What are the voices? And what am I? Am I part of some master plan or just another delusional mental patient? I am unsure what the future has in store for me, but I can confess I am a far different man compared to my breakdown. I care about people and am very sensitive emotionally. I hope I am a nicer person with strong morals, and I hope that the last twenty-eight years have made me wiser and more open-minded. These things are very important to me, as I feel I have some making up to do for my previous self.

Chapter Thirty-Six
Caring

Looking after my lovely wife is slowly taking its toll on my mental and physical health. I have been diagnosed with osteoarthritis in my hip and shoulder due to the heavy lifting. I am told I may need a new shoulder joint and will be seeing a surgeon in the near future. I do have the opportunity to use a hoist, but I am too impatient. The thing people don't realise about being an unpaid or even a paid carer is that it slowly burns you out. But I feel as though I cannot complain to anyone, as it is not me who is suffering. There are times I get so frustrated at just sitting down and being constantly asked for help. Occasionally, I would just like to shout out, *For the love of God, please leave me alone,* but of course, I can't. When I am struggling to cope, I try to put myself in Sam's shoes. I imagine myself in her wheelchair and being unable to get up and make a drink or walk in the garden for fresh air. When I think of her being in constant pain, I land with a bump and realise that I cannot complain.

There are times life becomes very mundane with the same routine day in day out, and life can seem like Groundhog Day for us both. I really do not mind wiping Sam's backside, and I try to make fun with it to lighten the mood for her. I get very silly and say things like, 'My God, this one is so big it has teeth', which always gets a laugh. Seeing my wife in pain is incredibly difficult; one day, for instance, as soon as I put Sam in her wheelchair, she went into a full body spasm. I gave her two antispasmodics, which did not work, and then a small dose of diazepam. After an hour and a half of Sam flaying around violently with her arms and torso, I called our doctor. He advised me to take her to hospital. I asked if I could give her another small dose of diazepam and he told me to go ahead. Within ten minutes, her spasms stopped, and she fell asleep. Diazepam/Valium is a muscle relaxant and can be used to sedate a patient or help with anxiety; it is not to be taken lightly, but thankfully it worked. Sam slept most of that day and was very groggy, but thankfully, the next day she was absolutely fine.

Showering can be a very difficult thing for us, as every time Sam gets in the shower, the water feels like sharp needles on her skin. After five minutes, she becomes so cold, her teeth chatter and she begins to cry. It is upsetting for me to witness this as I am rushing to get her dried and in a dressing gown, but I have learnt to switch off and get on with the job as compassionately and quickly as possible. I have to be hard sometimes because if I let her pain affect me, I become useless to her. But it is hard to switch off. Sam occasionally wets herself and suffers from pressure sores on her bottom. She has no feeling to go to the toilet for hours, but she will suddenly get a very strong urge to go and I do not always get her onto her commode in time. As a result, she pees in her clothes and on the floor. I found this very frustrating years ago, but I now figure getting frustrated or angry serves me no purpose, so I have let it go.

Some days I suffer from what is known as negative symptoms, which consists of lethargy, lack of motivation, and poor personal hygiene. Periods like this cycle make me feel quite wretched. My body feels incredibly heavy, and I ache all over like an old man. Days like these can be difficult caring, as I just want to curl up on the sofa, and often do. My family takes the mick out of me by saying I spend all my time on social media all day, which, to a certain extent, is true. The job is twenty-four hours a day with no day off except when our carers come in, so social media is like a window to the outside world. Our two ladies who care for Sam are a godsend. Once a week, they will take Sam out shopping for the afternoon, which gives her time away from me and the house. They also keep on top of the daily chores, such as ironing and cleaning, which become exhausting every day otherwise. They are both very hard workers and I have to force them to sit down and have a cuppa with us. They are both lovely company, and I like to think of them as extended family.

Chapter Thirty-Seven
Present Day

It is now December 2022, and we have recently begun making more friends over the last couple of years. We have been in Wales for six years now, and for the first time in a very long while, I am beginning to feel accepted. For my birthday, we had friends over, ordered Indian takeaway, played a nineties board game called Atmosphere, and got drunk. It feels like life is improving, and I've promised myself to make more of an effort with socialising.

I re-joined the Masons just over a year ago and I really enjoy the evenings out. They are a good bunch. I took up a sub officer position this year, so we regularly meet up to practise our words for lodge nights. Supper afterwards is always enjoyable. The Masons are the second biggest givers to charity after the National Lottery, which is something I'm really proud of. If you have ever been curious about the Masons, then look up Grand Lodge online and ask for more information. They are always looking for good men and will happily tell you more and help you join if you decide to.

My dad sold his house in Buckinghamshire and has bought a lovely two-bedroom bungalow in Surrey close to my sisters. I am glad that in his twilight years they will be there for him, and that he has his dream of a lovely bungalow with a nice garden to potter in. He isn't as fit as he used to be, so he has a lady in once a week to help him out.

Both of my sisters are happily married and have lovely children, and they've both done well in life.

My youngest son, Joshua, turned twenty this year. He is working as an apprentice electrician. He still lives at home and goes to college once a week to become qualified in three years. He is happy sitting and playing online games rather than going out and has just started playing *Eve Online* with me. My eldest son, Daniel, is just finishing his third year of university studying physical education and is hoping to sign up for teacher training afterwards. If Josh is an introvert, then Daniel is very much an extrovert. Considering their background, they have both done exceptionally well, and I am immensely proud of them both. I am looking forward to them both settling down and maybe gifting us some grandchildren.

Sam's mum became quite poorly many years ago with arthritis and fibromyalgia. She spends a lot of time sleeping and resting due to constant pain. She struggles to leave her bungalow and has become socially anxious. We try to visit, but if I'm honest, we do not visit enough. Ron, my father-in-law, does a sterling job caring for her and he keeps himself busy. In fact, he never stops. Ron visits as often as he can and has helped me a lot over the years, both with petty squabbles between Sam and me and things like laying a patio and putting a shed together. Sam's brother, Jay, moved in with his parents in Wales and is doing very well in a high-flying job, and he's met a nice girl.

My mum found out in 2021 that she had tongue cancer and fought very bravely. The pain relief she was given did not agree with her and made her hallucinate, and she could not eat, so she had to be fed with a bolus in her stomach. Towards the end, she suffered with terminal restlessness, and I was relieved when she passed away. I was also very angry at the end, because she just was not ready and I could not say what I wanted to say to her. My mum meant the world to me. Now I must try and be there for Sam and my kids just as she was there for me.

I do still hear voices, but not anywhere near as much. I also still get fatigued quite often, but life is so much better.

For the last three months I have been going to the gym with a buddy of mine three times a week, and although I don't notice much difference, I am toning up. Last year, I bought a bright-red Peugeot 205 1.9 CTI convertible which is great fun, driving with the hood down in the nice weather, Alison Limerick playing on the sound system.

Sam and I have had couples therapy, which has helped us both. It made me realise that the times when Sam is unhappy is not down to me, but that the nature of her disease frustrates her. I am her hands, and I am trying to learn to be more compassionate. We just need a really good holiday, two weeks in the sun, all-inclusive, getting drunk at night, and we will be fine.

I have no idea what the future brings, but I look forward to seeing increasingly light in the world.

The Succubus of Death

The Succubus of death sucks out your soul,

and leaves behind it a big gaping hole.

She will whip you and beat you and drive you insane.

Once in your life, you're never the same.

The Succubus of death will scream out your name,

as she clings to your life and eats at your brain;

she finds you somehow when you're at a loss,

and destroys your life without a toss.

The Succubus of death feeds off your pain,

until your world is over and starting to wane.

Then she will beat you as you kick and you scream,

and you're beginning to wonder, Is this a bad dream?

The Succubus of death has just one fear,

just as the end is beginning to draw near,

that you will find hope, and maybe love

and ask for forgiveness,

from Him up above.

Written by Darren Smith

Acknowledgements

I would like to thank everyone that has helped me publish my memoir. Primarily, my editor Claire Strombeck from Reedsy, whose words of encouragement and thorough diligence was second to none. She worked hard on my manuscript and answered all my questions with patience and grace. A huge thank you to Cleo Miele at Fiverr for her tireless work proofreading my manuscript. Cleo shocked me at how many errors I had made and promptly correctly them tirelessly. Thank you to Sharon Garrett from Sharon Garrett photography in Llandielo for her lovely photographs. Thank you to my sister Jennine for lending me the money to get this book self-published; it is surprising how much it all adds up. Thank you to polarbear19325 on fiverr for his thoroughly professional format of the interior of my book which looks amazing. Lastly thank you to Miblart for the book jacket design, her design was outstanding and more than I could expect. To Jason Elberts who patiently took and edited my picture for the front cover, thank you.

About the Author

Darren lives in an idyllic village in South Wales with the love of his life, his wife, Samantha. They have been together for twenty years and happily married for sixteen years. Darren has two cats and dotes on them both.

Darren spends too much time online and realises he needs to unplug and enjoy the real world more. He enjoys online gaming and MMORPGs. Although he enjoys classic two-stroke motorcycles, he realises he is probably too dangerous to be let loose on one in the foreseeable future. Darren loves driving his Peugeot 205 CTI around the lovely sweeping Welsh roads with the hood down, listening to Alison Limerick. Darren is very close to his family and loves large gatherings that involve silly board games and food.

If you enjoyed his book, please leave an honest review on Amazon and Goodreads – it would mean the world to him.

Darren would love to hear from you at dsmith3197@gmail.com, so drop him a line.

Printed in Great Britain
by Amazon